T0226911

# Collaborative Care of the Facial Injury Patient

*Guest Editors*

VIVEK SHETTY, DDS, Dr Med Dent
GRANT N. MARSHALL, PhD

## ORAL AND MAXILLOFACIAL SURGERY CLINICS OF NORTH AMERICA

www.oralmaxsurgery.theclinics.com

*Consulting Editor*
RICHARD H. HAUG, DDS

May 2010 • Volume 22 • Number 2

SAUNDERS an imprint of ELSEVIER, Inc.

**W.B. SAUNDERS COMPANY**
*A Division of Elsevier Inc.*

1600 John F. Kennedy Blvd. • Suite 1800 • Philadelphia, PA 19103-2899

www.oralmaxsurgery.theclinics.com

**ORAL AND MAXILLOFACIAL SURGERY CLINICS OF NORTH AMERICA Volume 22, Number 2**
**May 2010 ISSN 1042-3699, ISBN-13: 978-1-4377-1846-1**

Editor: John Vassallo; j.vassallo@elsevier.com

*Oral and Maxillofacial Surgery Clinics of North America* (ISSN 1042-3699) is published quarterly by Elsevier Inc., 360 Park Avenue South, New York, NY 10010-1710. Months of issue are February, May, August, and November. Business and Editorial Offices: 1600 John F. Kennedy Blvd., Suite 1800, Philadelphia, PA 19103-2899. Periodicals postage paid at New York, NY and additional mailing offices. Subscription prices are $304.00 per year for US individuals, $445.00 per year for US institutions, $140.00 per year for US students and residents, $351.00 per year for Canadian individuals, $530.00 per year for Canadian institutions, $405.00 per year for international individuals, $530.00 per year for international institutions and $190.00 per year for Canadian and foreign students/residents. To receive student/resident rate, orders must be accompanied by name or affiliated institution, date of term, and the *signature* of program/residency coordinator on institution letterhead. Orders will be billed at individual rate until proof of status is received. Foreign air speed delivery is included in all *Clinics* subscription prices. All prices are subject to change without notice. **POSTMASTER:** Send address changes to *Oral and Maxillofacial Surgery Clinics of North America,* Elsevier Periodicals Customer Service, 11830 Westline Industrial Drive, St. Louis, MO 63146. Tel: 1-800-654-2452 (U.S. and Canada); 314-447-8871 (outside U.S. and Canada). Fax: 314-447-8029. E-mail: journalscustomerservice-usa@elsevier.com (for print support); journalsonlinesupport-usa@elsevier.com (for online support).

*Reprints.* For copies of 100 or more, of articles in this publication, please contact the Commercial Reprints Department, Elsevier Inc., 360 Park Avenue South, New York, NY 10010-1710. Tel.: 212-633-3812; Fax: 212-462-1935; Email: reprints@elsevier.com.

*Oral and Maxillofacial Surgery Clinics of North America* is covered in MEDLINE/PubMed (*Index Medicus*).

Printed and bound by CPI Group (UK) Ltd, Croydon, CR0 4YY

Transferred to Digital Print 2011

# Contributors

## CONSULTING EDITOR

**RICHARD H. HAUG, DDS**
Carolinas Center for Oral Health
Charlotte, North Carolina

## GUEST EDITORS

**VIVEK SHETTY, DDS, Dr Med Dent**
Professor, Section of Oral and Maxillofacial
Surgery, UCLA School of Dentistry, University
of California, Los Angeles, Los Angeles,
California

**GRANT N. MARSHALL, PhD**
Health Program, Senior Behavioral Scientist,
RAND Corporation, Santa Monica, California

## AUTHORS

**MELANIE W. GIRONDA, PhD, MSW**
Adjunct Associate Professor, Division of Public
Health and Community Dentistry, School of
Dentistry, University of California, Los Angeles,
Los Angeles, California

**SHIRLEY M. GLYNN, PhD**
Clinical Research Psychologist, Research
Service, Veterans Affairs Greater Los Angeles
Healthcare System at West Los Angeles;
Research Psychologist, Semel Institute,
University of California, Los Angeles,
Los Angeles, California

**LESLIE R. HALPERN, DDS, MD, PhD, MPH**
Assistant Professor, Department of Oral and
Maxillofacial Surgery, Massachusetts General
Hospital, Harvard School of Dental Medicine,
Boston, Massachusetts

**ANNA LUI, MSW**
Department of Psychiatry, Veterans Affairs
Greater Los Angeles Healthcare System,
Los Angeles, California

**GRANT N. MARSHALL, PhD**
Health Program, Senior Behavorial Scientist,
RAND Corporation, Santa Monica,
California

**DEBRA A. MURPHY, PhD**
Research Psychologist, Health Risk Reduction
Projects, Integrated Substance Abuse
Programs, Department of Psychiatry,
University of California, Los Angeles,
Los Angeles, California

**MEGAN PETRIE, BA**
Research Study Coordinator, Department of
Psychiatry and Behavioral Sciences, University
of Washington, Seattle, Washington

**VIVEK SHETTY, DDS, Dr Med Dent**
Professor, Section of Oral and Maxillofacial
Surgery, UCLA School of Dentistry, University of
California, Los Angeles, Los Angeles, California

**EUNICE C. WONG, PhD**
Associate Behavioral Scientist, RAND
Corporation, Santa Monica, California

**MASAKI YAMAGUCHI, PhD**
Professor, Department of Welfare
Engineering, Faculty of Engineering,
Iwate University, Ueda, Morioka City, Japan

**DOUGLAS ZATZICK, MD**
Associate Professor, Department
of Psychiatry and Behavioral Sciences,
University of Washington, Seattle,
Washington

# Contents

Individuals with orofacial injury presenting to urban trauma centers in the United States tend to be disproportionately socioeconomically disadvantaged, young, adult, ethnic minority men. Most injuries are assaultive in origin, suggesting poor impulse control and maladaptive social behaviors. Compared with matched control populations, patients with orofacial injuries are more likely to report higher levels of substance use behaviors and to manifest greater levels of hostility, anxiety, and depression. Although they have significantly greater current and lifetime need for mental health service and social service, actual use of social services is low. The underlying psychosocial characteristics of many patients with orofacial injury, along with unmet service needs, render them vulnerable for posttrauma psychological sequelae and may compromise functional outcomes and recovery.

Significant subsets of patients who experience orofacial injury are at risk for developing adverse psychological sequelae such as posttraumatic stress disorder and depression. If undetected and untreated, the psychopathology can become recalcitrant and burden the social and vocational functioning of the patients and greatly diminish their quality of life. The hospital encounter and follow-up care visits provide the oral and maxillofacial surgeon with opportunities to screen for emerging psychological problems. Several screening instruments are available to assist the surgeon in identifying individuals who are at risk for subsequent mental health problems. Facilitated referrals to mental health services can be a practical approach for improving comprehensive medical care for vulnerable individuals and for reducing the potential morbidity of these covert, but disabling, sequelae.

After facial trauma, a subset of patients develops mental health problems, particularly posttraumatic stress disorder (PTSD) and major depression. Early identification of patients who may be at risk for these disorders can facilitate referral for further psychiatric evaluation and possible treatment. Brief, easy-to-use screening tools are available to assist in the process of recognizing these individuals. This article provides a review of some of the most commonly used short screeners for PTSD and major depression. Incorporating information gleaned from these self-administered screeners into the routine evaluation of patients with facial trauma will help to address the mental health needs that are associated with orofacial injury.

Substance use is a major contributing factor to the interpersonal violence that accounts for a significant proportion of facial injuries among adults and adolescents;

thus, violence is the main "pathway" through which substance use and injuries are linked. Beyond causality, substance use continues to influence recovery from the injury through its impact on the healing process (eg, patient noncompliance, suppression of T-cell counts, susceptibility to bacterial colonization, and protein production). Further exacerbating this issue are significant rates of injury recidivism and the lack of motivation to seek treatment for underlying substance-use problems. As a frontline care provider, the oral and maxillofacial surgeon has a responsibility to screen and refer patients for any needed specialty treatment (including substance-use treatment, violence reduction, and posttraumatic stress reduction). Recognizing and addressing these issues requires a paradigm shift that involves integration of multidisciplinary expertise.

Health care professionals have increasingly recognized that intimate partner violence (IPV) is a highly prevalent public health problem with devastating effects on individuals, families, and communities. However, there are no obvious clinical characteristics of IPV. Interventions may prevent future IPV-related injuries, but they cannot be initiated until the diagnosis is made. Because of the frequency of IPV-related orofacial injuries, oral and maxillofacial surgeons (OMSs) may be the first and only health care providers to see these patients. Therefore, OMSs are in a pivotal position to diagnosis IPV-related injuries and expedite referral for interventional therapy. This article presents data that support the use of orofacial injuries as a prime predictor variable in identifying victims of IPV and provides: (1) an overview of the epidemiology of IPV-related orofacial injuries; (2) a discussion of the role of head, neck, and facial injuries as markers of IPV, and their role as a diagnostic tool to facilitate the early diagnosis and referral for management of IPV; (3) a list of the advantages and limitations of using orofacial injuries as indicators of IPV; and (4) future directions to improve efforts to educate OMSs in identifying patients who are at high risk for an IPV-related injury.

Collaborative care interventions show significant promise in facilitating integrative care, which addresses the physical and mental health needs of patients with orofacial trauma. Ensuring the successful implementation of collaborative care interventions depends on having an adequate understanding of the potential barriers to the provision and receipt of mental health services within specific clinical settings. This article reviews recent findings on the patients' and providers' perceptions of barriers to psychosocial aftercare services in oral and maxillofacial trauma care settings. These findings indicate that although patients and providers recognize the need for psychosocial aftercare, they report substantial barriers to these services. Structural barriers, such as not knowing where to obtain services and financial cost, are the major obstacles among patients. Among providers, structural barriers also serve as significant impediments to the provision of psychosocial services. Some of the most common structural barriers reported by providers include a shortage of financial resources, trained clinical staff, and space. Although collaborative care interventions may be well suited to capitalize on patients' and providers' interests in psychosocial aftercare programs, further research is needed to determine the viability of this promising aftercare model within oral and maxillofacial trauma care settings.

Although many trauma centers provide excellent surgical care, little attention is paid to psychosocial needs and problems of posttrauma adaptation. Social support and resource needs have been identified as significant mediators of recovery after injuries. This article presents an overview of various social and material resources instrumental to psychological adjustment and recovery. It also discusses the ways in which complex social networks can be both beneficial and damaging toward the recovery process and the implications for clinical care of patients with orofacial injury. Finally, appropriate social support resource measuring tools that may be used in clinical settings are presented.

Collaborative care is a disease management strategy that aims to simultaneously target medical/surgical (eg, physical injury) and psychiatric (eg, posttraumatic stress disorder [PTSD] and depression) conditions. Collaborative care interventions hold promise for the delivery of mental health interventions in acute care as they can incorporate frontline trauma center providers, such as social workers and nurses, into early mental health services delivery and can link trauma center care to outpatient services. Initial randomized clinical trial evidence suggests that collaborative care interventions that incorporate evidence-based motivational interviewing targeting alcohol use, as well as pharmacotherapy and psychotherapy targeting PTSD, may reduce both alcohol and PTSD symptoms among injured trauma surgery patients. Trials conducted to date thus suggest that early mental health interventions can be feasibly and effectively delivered from trauma centers. Future collaborative care investigations that refine routine acute care treatment procedures and target acute care policy mandates can improve the quality of mental health care for Americans injured in the wake of individual and mass trauma.

After facial trauma, a distinct subset of patients goes on to develop mental health problems including recalcitrant psychopathology. Early identification of maladaptive stress reactions provides opportunities for initiating preemptive mental health interventions and hinges on the surgeon's ability to differentiate between transient distress and precursors of recalcitrant psychiatric sequelae. The comprehensive care of injured patients will benefit greatly from objective adjuncts and decision-making tools to complement the clinical evaluation. This article addresses meeting the need for practical, standardized, and reliable screening strategies through promising developments in the use of stress response biomarkers and biosensing technology. The systematic interrogation of differentially expressed stress response biomarkers in saliva now permits rapid assessment of the psychopathogical response to the stressor. Quantitative, point-of-use measurements of the traumatic stress response will greatly improve the nosology of posttraumatic stress disorders and help advance the screening, diagnosis, treatment, and prevention of mental health consequences of violence and trauma.

# Oral and Maxillofacial Surgery Clinics of North America

## THE CLINICS ARE NOW AVAILABLE ONLINE!

Access your subscription at:
**www.theclinics.com**

# Preface
# Collaborative Care of the Facial Injury Patient

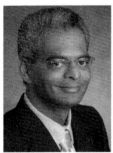
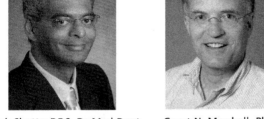

Vivek Shetty, DDS, Dr Med Dent     Grant N. Marshall, PhD

*Guest Editors*

Intentional injury persists as a major challenge to trauma centers, exerting its greatest impact on socioeconomically marginalized populations. Beyond the substantial burden of disease with respect to economic cost and human suffering, the intentional nature of the injury renders it a major risk factor for reinjury. Most of these injuries tend to derive from impulsive actions, often against a background of recent substance use, alcoholism, severe stress, or psychosocial–behavioral difficulties. In many instances, the traumatic stressor sets the stage for subsequent psychosocial sequelae that can be as disabling as any physical handicap, negatively affecting recovery and quality of life.

As a distinct entity of the spectrum of injuries, orofacial injury is worthy of special emphasis because it occurs with high frequency,[1] disproportionately affects vulnerable populations,[2,3] involves an anatomic region that largely defines perceptions of self-image and identity,[4] is often associated with persistent disabilities, and uses up the majority of dental/oral surgical services provided by public hospitals.[3,5] Because the facial region is a particular target in aggravated assault,[6,7] injury to the head and neck region is regarded as a prominent clinical sign of interpersonal violence and, especially in women, is posited as a marker of intimate partner violence (see article by Leslie R. Halpern elsewhere in this issue for further explanation of this topic). Given

the centrality of the face to physical and psychosocial functioning, injuries to this part of the body can be traumatic and stressful.[8–11] Because the consequences of orofacial injury can extend beyond an impairment of normal eating habits to have an impact on an individual's perceptions of self-image and identity, adjustment to a facial disability can be more troublesome than an extremity problem.[12] As Glynn and Shetty point out in this issue, the underlying psychosocial characteristics of many orofacial injury patients render them especially vulnerable to posttrauma psychological sequelae and significant subsets end up manifesting acute and long-term psychopathology, such as posttraumatic stress disorder (PTSD) and major depression.

Of the various antecedent behaviors associated with injury, substance (alcohol/illicit drug) use is one of the most prevalent (see article by Debra A. Murphy elsewhere in this issue for further explanation of this topic). Coping with the traumatic event and its aftermath poses a special dilemma in patients whose alcohol/drug use may have contributed to their orofacial injury. Substance use is a common avoidance response to traumatic injury and may serve as a type of self-medication of anxiety and depressive symptoms.[13] In an attempt to deal with traumatic hyperarousal, which interferes with sleep, individuals may use or escalate the use of alcohol or illicit drugs. The negative social consequences of alcohol/drug use—which include

Oral Maxillofacial Surg Clin N Am 22 (2010) ix–xii
doi:10.1016/j.coms.2010.02.001

involvement in arguments and fights; loss of employment and broken relationships; and legal problems, such as arrests for abuse, possession, or selling of illicit drugs—only compound the adverse psychological consequences of traumatic injury.

The consequences of untreated substance abuse and antecedent risk behaviors are just as serious. Rivara and colleagues[14] found that trauma center patients who screened positive for alcoholism were 3.5 times more likely than other patients to be readmitted for a second injury episode. The evidence linking substance use and injury is so strong that many investigators have argued for treating trauma center admission as a secondary symptom of an underlying substance abuse problem, proposing that any efforts to reduce the risk of injury recurrence are unlikely to be successful if the underlying problem is not addressed.[15–18] Following up on the strong suggestion of causality, several national agencies, including the Institute of Medicine,[19] the Centers for Disease Control and Prevention, the Substance Abuse and Mental Health Services Administration,[20] and the US Department of Health and Human Services,[21] have recommended that all trauma patients be screened for substance use and referrals made to appropriate treatment programs matched to the intensity of the patient's problem.

The multifaceted physical, social, and psychological problems affecting many survivors of facial trauma provide a compelling argument for extending trauma care beyond repair of the physical injury to an integrated, multispecialty approach addressing attendant risk behaviors and comorbidities. The trauma center is often the only contact with the health care system for orofacial injury victims, the majority of whom tend to be young and otherwise healthy. For such patients, the hospital encounter provides a window of opportunity for detecting and referral for treatment of any antecedent risky behaviors as well as emerging psychosocial sequelae. Brief screening strategies within the context of surgical care could be used to identify those patients who have, or are at risk for, problem behaviors or psychological problems. Targeted referrals to allied services would allow comprehensive management approaches and an appropriate focusing of the limited time and resources typical of trauma care settings.

The article by Murphy (elsewhere in this issue) summarizes some brief and focused substance use screening strategies that make it possible to identify individuals at risk for hazardous drinking or drug use and who are most likely to benefit from referral and intervention. Similarly, Marshall's article (elsewhere in this issue) summarizes instruments that could be used for early identification of individuals who develop posttraumatic stress reactions, such as major depression or PTSD, secondary to their facial injury. Although formal diagnosis of these conditions requires a detailed psychiatric interview, these brief screening tools can assist surgeons in screening patients and facilitating referral to mental health specialists for treatment or a more through diagnostic examination. Gironda and Lui (elsewhere in this issue) describe how resource needs moderate the impact of the traumatic stressor and suggest how social support can be harnessed as a resource to facilitate recovery from violence-related facial injury.

The availability of systems to address the multifaceted service needs of injured patients is only one part of the collaborative care approach—patients must also be willing and able to use these services. Wong and Marshall (elsewhere in this issue) synthesize the available research literature concerning perceived barriers to the use of psychosocial aftercare programs by persons with violence-related orofacial injury. In identifying salient barriers to comprehensive care, they underscore the receptiveness of patients to psychosocial aftercare programs and the tendency of surgeons to underestimate their influence in affecting patient use of such programs. As discussed by Petrie and Zatzick (elsewhere in this issue), collaborative care models involving the closely integrated collaboration of multiple specialists have proved efficacious in general trauma settings. These collaborative care interventions, which attempt to address the full range of physical, mental, psychosocial, and other problems experienced by injury survivors, have potential usefulness in the care of facial injury patients. Equally promising are emerging portable technologies that can be used by surgeons as adjunctive aids to facilitate point-of-care, biomarker-based screening and identification of psychological comorbidy. Shetty and Yamaguchi (elsewhere in this issue) describe their development of handheld biosensors for systematic interrogation of differentially expressed stress response biomarkers in saliva and their potential application in assessing an individual's psychological response to the traumatic stressor.

All too often, restitution of the overt physical injury is considered the endpoint of facial injury care. Even when an underlying problem is suspected, the process of screening and referral for needed treatment or intervention is haphazard and highly fragmented. Current care of facial injury patients is notable for a general lack of involvement of other health care professionals, such as psychologists, substance abuse counselors, and social workers. Drawing on the research experiences and specialty insights of a multidisciplinary team of contributors, this issue of the *Oral and Maxillofacial Surgery Clinics of North America* provides a rationale and framework for comprehensive care of patients presenting with orofacial injury. To make a positive impact on the orofacial injury problem, care of injured patients needs to be expanded beyond a patient's immediate surgical needs to involve consideration of the underlying causes of injury and potential nonphysical sequelae. The continuing inability to synthesize essential patient needs into a collaborative and interdisciplinary response has tremendous consequences for injured patients. An increased awareness of the psychosocial antecedents and consequences of orofacial injury is an important first step toward providing the comprehensive care needed by many patients with facial injury and we offer this issue as a stimulus.

## ACKNOWLEDGMENTS

This issue of the *Oral and Maxillofacial Surgery Clinics of North America* was made possible by support from the National Institutes of Health - National Institute on Drug Abuse (NIH-NIDA) which funded major parts of the research upon which this issue is based. Its contents are solely the responsibility of the authors and do not necessarily represent the official views of NIH or NIDA.

Vivek Shetty, DDS, Dr Med Dent
Section of Oral and Maxillofacial Surgery
23-009 UCLA School of Dentistry
10833 Le Conte Avenue
Los Angeles, CA 90095-1668, USA

Grant N. Marshall, PhD
RAND Corporation, 1776 Main Street
Santa Monica, CA 90407, USA

E-mail addresses:
vshetty@ucla.edu (V. Shetty)
grantm@rand.org (G.N. Marshall)

## REFERENCES

1. Mathog RH, Toma V, Clayman L, et al. Nonunion of the mandible: an analysis of contributing factors. J Oral Maxillofac Surg 2000;58(7):746–52.
2. Hall SC, Ofodile PA. Mandibular fractures in an American inner city: the Harlem Hospital Center experience. J Natl Med Assoc 1991;83:421–3.
3. Leathers R, Shetty V, Black E, et al. Orofacial injury profiles and patterns of care in an inner city hospital. Int J Oral Biology 1998;23:53–8.
4. Bronheim H, Strain JJ, Biller HF. Psychiatric aspects of head and neck surgery. Part II: body image and psychiatric intervention. Gen Hosp Psychiatry 1991;13(4):225–32.
5. Leathers R, Le AD, Black E, et al. Orofacial injury in underserved minority populations. Dent Clin North Am 2003;47(1):127–39.
6. Telfer MR, Jones GM, Shepherd JR. Trends in the etiology of maxillofacial fractures in the United Kingdom. Br J Oral Maxillofac Surg 1991;29:250–5.
7. Waller JA, Skelly JM, Davis JH. Characteristics, costs and effects of violence in Vermont. J Trauma 1994;37:921–7.
8. Glynn SM, Asarnow JR, Asarnow R, et al. The development of acute post-traumatic stress disorder after orofacial injury: a prospective study in a large urban hospital. J Oral Maxillofac Surg 2003;61(7): 785–92.
9. Glynn SM, Shetty V, Elliot-Brown K, et al. Chronic posttraumatic stress disorder after facial injury: a 1-year prospective cohort study. J Trauma 2007; 62(2):410–8 [discussion: 418].
10. Lento J, Glynn S, Shetty V, et al. Psychologic functioning and needs of indigent patients with facial injury: a prospective controlled study. J Oral Maxillofac Surg 2004;62(8):925–32.
11. Shetty V, Dent DM, Glynn S, et al. Psychosocial sequelae and correlates of orofacial injury. Dent Clin North Am 2003;47(1):141–57, xi.
12. Wright BA. Physical disability: a psychosocial approach. 2nd edition. New York: Harper & Row, Publishers Inc; 1990.
13. Bremner JD, Southwick SM, Darnell A, et al. Chronic PTSD in Vietnam combat veterans: course of illness and substance abuse. Am J Psychiatry 1996;153(3): 369–75.
14. Rivara FP, Koepsell TD, Jurkovich GJ, et al. The effects of alcohol abuse on readmission for trauma. JAMA 1993;270:1962–4.
15. Clark DE, McCarthy E, Robinson E. Trauma as a symptom of alcoholism. Ann Emerg Med 1985; 14(3):274–80.
16. Rivara FP, Mueller BA, Fligner CL, et al. Drug use in trauma victims. J Trauma 1989;29(4): 462–70.
17. Cherpital CJ. Alcohol and injuries: a review of international emergency room studies. Addiction 1993; 88:923–93.
18. Cherpital CJ. Alcohol consumption among emergency room patients: Comparison of county/ community hospitals and an HMO. J Stud Alcohol 1993;54:432–40.
19. Institute of Medicine. National Academy of Sciences. Broadening the base of treatment for

alcohol problems. Washington, DC: National Academy Press; 1990.

20. Substance Abuse and Mental Health Services Administration. Alcohol, and other drug screening of hospitalized trauma patients. Rockville (MD): Substance Abuse and Mental Health Services Administration, (DHHS publication No (SMA) 95-3041); 1995.

21. U.S. Department of Health and Human Services. Model trauma care plan. Rockville (MD): DHHS; 1992.

# The Psychosocial Characteristics and Needs of Patients Presenting with Orofacial Injury

Shirley M. Glynn, PhD[a,b,*]

## KEYWORDS

- Sociodemographic • Socioeconomic
- Orofacial injury • Trauma

Although maxillofacial fractures are one of the more common types of injuries treated at trauma centers, the surgical literature is largely confined to reporting the epidemiology of these injuries or to articulating practice guidelines. The current practice of viewing these injuries only within a surgical context tends to ignore equally salient features that can and do affect the health outcomes. Over the past decade, the efforts of a small group of investigators[1–3] have increasingly sensitized the surgical community to the hidden social and psychological factors that adversely influence treatment response and increase the risk of recidivism or reinjury. Orofacial injuries are becoming understood as occurring within an identifiable interpersonal and intrapersonal context.[4] Providing effective surgical care is a critical aspect of recovery, but so is meeting the concurrent social and psychological needs of patients that may render them at particular risk for poor psychosocial adjustment after the traumatic event. Untreated emotional and behavioral disorders, including depression and antisocial behavior problems, contribute to poor overall social functioning, occupational failure, substance abuse, and continuing risking behaviors that increase the risk of violence and reinjury. This recognition provides the basis for a model of coordinated care, wherein the surgeons work together with other specialists to develop and implement a comprehensive and integrated treatment plan that addresses the physical and the psychosocial needs of the patient with orofacial injury.

The preceding articles and several studies using archival data have summarized the sociodemographic characteristics of persons presenting with maxillofacial fractures to trauma centers. Most patients, particularly those treated at inner city hospitals, tend to be young men who sustain injuries as a result of interpersonal violence. A retrospective review[5] of 267 patients treated for orofacial injury at a level 1 trauma unit in Washington, DC, found that the patients were predominantly men (86%) and mostly (37%) young adults between 25 and 34 years. Nearly 79% of the injuries resulted from interpersonal violence, and illicit substance use at the time of trauma was reported in 55% of cases. Scherer and colleagues,[6] who reviewed the hospital records of all 788 patients who presented with facial fractures to a Detroit-based trauma center, reported similar profiles. The injured population was predominantly male (80.9%) and

This work was supported by Grant Number P50/DE-10598 from the National Institutes of Health/National Institute of Dental and Craniofacial Research.

[a] Research Service, VA Greater Los Angeles Healthcare System at West Los Angeles, B151J, 11301 Wilshire Boulevard, Los Angeles, CA 90073, USA
[b] Semel Institute, University of California, Los Angeles, CA, USA
* Research Service, VA Greater Los Angeles Healthcare System, West Los Angeles, B151J, 11301 Wilshire Boulevard, Los Angeles, CA 90073.
E-mail address: sglynn@ucla.edu

Oral Maxillofacial Surg Clin N Am 22 (2010) 209–215
doi:10.1016/j.coms.2010.01.003
1042-3699/10/$ – see front matter. Published by Elsevier Inc.

African American (71.6%), with assault with a fist or blunt object (70.1%) being the most frequent cause of injury. Although these data highlight the association of sociodemographic and interpersonal variables with orofacial injuries, they largely ignore the broader social and psychological factors that led to these injuries or their influence on patient recovery. These social and psychological factors and their influence are discussed in this article.

Three research teams across the United States, the University of California, Los Angeles (UCLA)[4–7]; the Medical College of Virginia, Richmond[7]; and the University of Medicine and Dentistry of New Jersey (UMDNJ)[8]; and the University of California, Los Angeles (UCLA),[9–10] have recently reported data emphasizing the social and psychological characteristics of persons presenting for care of their facial injuries (most typically, mandible fractures). In contrast to the archival reports mentioned earlier, these newer studies were designed to collect data prospectively, and with particular attention paid to obtaining contextual social and psychological data from the patients. The objectives of these studies include determining injury risk factors and predictors of outcomes and potential need for other care. All of these prospective studies involve predominantly socioeconomically disadvantaged, ethnically diverse populations in urban settings. In this article, the author compares and contrasts the findings of these clinical research teams concerning the sociodemographic and psychological factors present at the time of injury or during the early days of recovery. Firstly, the similarities in demographics among the samples in these studies are noted. Secondly, published data are presented to highlight social and psychological factors associated with orofacial injury. Thirdly, comparison data between those with orofacial injury and noninjured, sociodemographically matched controls[9] are described to distinguish personal from environmental factors, which may be related to risk of injury. Lastly, the implications of the findings as they pertain to collaborative care models that address the psychosocial aspects in addition to the physical injury are discussed. The overall intent here is to highlight the demographic, social, and psychological factors that may affect care and subsequent recovery of persons who experience orofacial trauma. Focus is on perioperative factors that are apparent or readily elicited at the time of the initial patient encounter or in the early recovery period rather than on factors such as the development of anxiety disorders or loss of social support, which may manifest long after the surgical follow-up has ended. The long-term psychosocial sequelae are discussed in subsequent articles. The underlying premise is that by viewing patients in a broader context at the initial encounter, clinicians will be able to see beyond the physical injury to include consideration of equally pernicious psychosocial factors that can prevent comprehensive patient recovery or set the stage for recurrent injury.

## SOCIODEMOGRAPHIC PROFILES OF PATIENTS WITH OROFACIAL INJURY

Sample sizes in the cohorts investigated prospectively by the various research groups range from 47 at the Medical College of Virginia[7] to 92 at UMDNJ[8] to 336 at UCLA.[9] In 2 of the research studies, at UCLA and at UMDNJ, investigators approached consecutive admissions seeking care for an orofacial injury (typically a mandibular fracture); such a recruitment strategy reduces bias and likely increases the generalizability of findings. The strategy for recruitment into the study at the Medical College of Virginia is not clear. In the UCLA studies,[2,9,10] patients were approached in the emergency department or shortly thereafter at an early follow-up appointment. The participants at the Medical College of Virginia were approached during an early follow-up appointment, whereas it is unclear how soon after the injury participants were enrolled in the UMDNJ study. Causes of the injury were not systematically reported in the samples.

Overall, affected subjects were primarily men (mean percentage range from 78.7%–89.9%); the subjects were typically in their late 20s to early 30s (mean age range from 29–35 years). All studies except the one at UMDNJ reported the ethnic compositions of their samples. In the study at Medical College of Virginia, African Americans predominated. The UCLA-based studies showed a preponderance of African American and Hispanic subjects. The rates of unemployment ranged from 60% to 67.4% in the UCLA studies; the employment status was not reported for the other 2 samples. Similarly, marital status was available only in the samples from UCLA; approximately 75% of the participants were then single. Taken together, these data suggest that the typical person presenting for urgent care of an orofacial injury is a socioeconomically disadvantaged, young ethnic minority male, who is at present unmarried. These data are consistent with those from earlier retrospective studies.[5,6]

## PSYCHOSOCIAL NEEDS OF INJURED PATIENTS

The sociodemographic description given earlier suggests a preexisting financial stress and lack of social support in many individuals presenting for care of a mandibular fracture. However, the reports from the 3 research centers (UCLA, Virginia, and UMDNJ) show additional social needs and psychological issues in many injured individuals around the time of the injury or in the immediate recovery period. Although these variables have been assessed in different ways, the themes emerging from these studies suggest that patients with orofacial injuries have a complicated set of needs and concerns impinging on them at the time of their injury and that they are interested in obtaining assistance if it were available to them.

The association of alcohol with injury has long been acknowledged in trauma research, and alcohol consumption is a major etiologic factor in intentional and unintentional trauma.[11] In their cohort of patients with orofacial injury, Auerbach and colleagues[7] at the Medical College in Virginia found that 36% of the patients had scores on the Alcohol Use Disorders Identification Test,[12] which indicates "hazardous and harmful alcohol use, as well as possible alcohol dependence." From the UCLA group, Wong and colleagues[13] reported that 31% of their injured sample with posttraumatic stress disorder (PTSD) met screening criteria for probable alcohol use disorder by using the Rapid Alcohol Problem Screen[14] (see the article by Murphy elsewhere in this issue for greater discussion of substance use issues). The care providers also recognized the prominence of substance use problems in patients with orofacial injury.[15] In a different UCLA cohort, Glynn and colleagues[2] found that the responses to the commonly used CAGE questionnaire suggested a possible alcohol problem in 62% of the subjects.[16] These estimates are all markedly higher than the prevalence rates of alcohol problems found in African American (6.92%) and Hispanic (9.08%) men in their 20s, which was found in a recently published large-scale national epidemiologic study.[17] The drug use patterns, in contrast to alcohol use patterns, were not systematically investigated in these samples. Because drug and alcohol use often co-occur, it is likely that even more injured persons would have been identified as having likely substance use issues if drug use patterns had been systematically queried in these studies.

A history of prior trauma seems common in patients with orofacial injuries. At UMDNJ,[8] 42.4% of the sample reported previous injuries; among those, most of the patients (59%) had experienced assault. Patients previously assaulted were 1.5 times more likely to report assault as the cause of their current orofacial injury. In the

UCLA sample, Glynn and colleagues[2] found that 85.1% of the patients had experienced a prior traumatic event, as operationalized on the exposure items of the Posttraumatic Stress Diagnosis Scale.[18] The rates of prior trauma exposure reported in the UMDNJ and UCLA samples are comparable to those reported in large-scale studies of ethnically diverse samples.[19,20] The rate of prior PTSD reported in the UCLA sample, as indicated by self-report of symptoms, was slightly higher (14.5%) than the rates typically reported in larger epidemiologic studies (8%–12%).[19,21]

High rates of prior trauma exposure, alcohol use, and unemployment or underemployment, coupled with the burden of an acute orofacial injury are the reasons behind a substantial proportion of the injured participants seeming open to the possibility of receiving some type of social service or mental health treatment as part of the care of their orofacial injury. In the UCLA sample,[9] participants were first queried about their lifetime and current perceived need and use of social service and mental health services, using the Service Use and Adjustment Problem Screen (SUAPS).[22] This brief self-report screening tool included 11 items focusing on mental health and social service problems and use. Specific areas assessed included mental health problems, suicide attempts, alcohol use problems, drug use problems, impairment, problems with the law, problems with employment (fired or laid off), school expulsion or multiple suspensions, mental health and substance abuse treatment, and homelessness. Individuals are asked to indicate whether they experienced this situation during their lifetimes. Response options included (1) no, (2) yes, during the past year, (3) yes, but not during the past year, and (4) yes, in the past year and before. Responses are summed to provide an index of (1) any self-identified mental health need, (2) any self-identified service need, and (3) any service use. Overall, 78.3% of the sample indicated a lifetime social service need and 53% indicated a lifetime mental health need, with 48.6% indicating a current social service need and 36.9% indicating a current mental health need at the time of the incident. Despite this need, current service use rates were only 11.3%.

Recognition of this need for either some change in behavior or engagement in collaborative care was reflected in the UCLA and UMDNJ samples. To assess participant interest in an aftercare program specifically designed to address reported mental health problems, Wong and colleagues[13] queried a cohort of UCLA subjects to ascertain their interest in a program designed to help assist them with anxiety, depression, and alcohol problems. Responses were provided on a 3-point scale ranging from 1 (very interested) to 3 (not at all interested). Participants screened (facial injury with a likely diagnosis of PTSD, depression, or an alcohol use disorder) achieved a mean score of 1.68, suggesting at least a moderate interest in aftercare. However, many barriers to accessing treatment were identified by participants[13] and their care providers,[15] with the primary barriers being lack of information on suitable programs, cost, transportation, and other competing responsibilities of the care providers. At UMDNJ, Laski and colleagues[8] incorporated the transtheoretical stages of change model[23] to understand the receptivity of participants to attending a workshop to reduce risk of reexposure to violence. The transtheoretical stages of change model proposes that individuals pass through predictable stages when improving health behaviors: precontemplation (no active consideration of change), contemplation (consideration of change, but no current commitment to change), preparation (active commitment to change but not taking action yet), action (specific actions currently being engaged in to bring about the behavior change), and maintenance/relapse (behavior change has or has not been achieved for at least 6 months). Most orofacially injured participants in the Laski study were in the contemplation (54%) or preparation stage (28%) to enter a violence reduction program if it were offered. These results suggest that if individuals are approached around the time of injury, they may be especially amenable to address problematic behaviors that continue to put them at risk.

The results of these studies suggest that individuals presenting with orofacial injury seem to be at an increased risk of concurrent alcohol use problems and may have had prior traumatic exposure. Most have experienced prior social service and mental health needs in their lives, and 35% to 45% are experiencing this need around the time of injury, although actual service use rates are low. Although there seems to be a willingness to consider professional intervention among injury survivors, perceived access is a significant obstacle. These results highlight the multidimensional nature of the obstacles that many injured patients must overcome to achieve high levels of physical and social functioning.

## PATIENTS WITH OROFACIAL INJURY DIFFER FROM THEIR MATCHED, UNINJURED COHORTS

Socioeconomically disadvantaged individuals tend to be disproportionately affected by facial trauma.[24] One challenge to understanding the characteristics of the orofacial injury samples discussed to this point is that many participants were from economically deprived areas and lived under extreme social and environmental stress. This pattern of findings raises the question of whether the risk factors highlighted here result primarily from economic deprivation or whether they are more specific personal characteristics predisposing individuals to an orofacial injury. There are few norms with which we can compare the results obtained in these trials to clarify this issue. Are the social and psychological problems associated with assault-related orofacial injury uniquely associated with this group or are the problems generally consistent with the socioeconomic milieu in which these patients find themselves?

The data collected as part of a prospective study conducted by the UCLA group[9] help distinguish the relative importance of social and economic deprivation from other factors that contribute to the risk of orofacial injury and adverse outcomes. Apart from the cohort of 336 orofacial injury patients, similar demographic, social history, and psychological functioning data were collected from 119 patients presenting for elective third molar extractions. Being drawn from the same urban environment, the third molar extraction group served as a control for the larger economic and social context of the injured individuals. Using assessment measures described earlier, sociodemographic data, information on alcohol use obtained from the CAGE questionnaire, and data on prior trauma exposure were collected from both groups. A widely used measure of psychological distress and psychiatric complaints, the Brief Symptom Inventory (BSI),[25] was also used. The BSI is a brief, multidimensional self-report assessment consisting of 53 items in 9 dimensions. For purposes of this study, the anxiety, depression, phobic anxiety, hostility, and obsessive-compulsive scales were used. The patients rated each item on a 5-point scale of distress from 0 (not at all) to 4 (extremely). Only raw scores were used in the analysis because the study sample substantially differed from the ethnic distribution of the normative sample used to generate the standardized scores for the BSI. Patients from both the groups also completed the SUAPS, described earlier, which assessed social and mental health service need and use, lifetime and current. These data were all collected on admission or within 10 days of the injury or surgical extraction.

Even within the same socioeconomic urban setting, the injured and third molar extraction samples differed in significant ways. The third molar extraction group was composed of significantly more women (25.2% vs 12.1%), tended to be younger (55.5% in the 18- to 29-year age group vs 38.8%), and was less likely to report any alcohol use (32.8% vs 17.3% abstinent) or any drug use (71.4% vs 51.1% no drug use). Thus, even within an identical environmental context, in comparison with those having an elective third molar extraction, individuals suffering a facial injury were found to be mostly men, to be slightly older, and to be using alcohol or drugs. However, the samples did not differ in marital status (<20% in each sample were married), ethnicity (more than 60% were African American in both groups), education (more than 60% had at least graduated from high school in both groups), or employment (more than over 60% were unemployed in both groups). In a follow-up study of similar patients (n = 98) with mandibular fractures and a comparison group of third molar extraction patients (n = 103), Atchison and colleagues[26] noted that the patients with facial injury also reported less perceived social support and smaller social networks.

Differences in psychological and social variables in these 2 samples were then examined after adjusting statistically for preexisting differences in the sociodemographic composition of the 2 groups. Ten days postinjury, the injured group showed significantly more depression, anxiety, hostility, and phobic anxiety on the BSI as well as significantly more need for current and lifetime mental health and social service. The higher rates of anxiety and depression in the injury group compared with the third molar extraction cohort is striking, given that the extraction group consisted of more women than the orofacial injury group. Women are typically associated with greater self-reported rates of depression[27] and most anxiety disorders,[28] and thus we might have expected a greater preponderance of these symptoms in the comparison group. However, there were no differences in the obsessive-compulsive symptoms or current or lifetime social service use between the 2 groups. These results suggest that, even in an economically disadvantaged, ethnically diverse population, individuals at risk for severe orofacial injury exhibit identifiable psychological characteristics.

## CLINICAL IMPLICATIONS

There is a remarkable consistency in the findings of the studies reviewed here on factors associated with sustaining a severe orofacial injury such as a mandibular fracture and presenting for treatment at a large urban hospital. Injured patients were typically unemployed, socially disadvantaged, ethnic

minority men in their mid-20s to their mid-30s. They had likely been exposed to prior traumatic events, although they typically did not have PTSD from these events at the time of the orofacial injury. Most of the orofacial injuries resulted from assaults, and alcohol or substance use was often involved. Injured subjects evidenced greater levels of substance and/or alcohol use, less perceived social support and smaller social networks, as well as higher rates of depression, anxiety, and hostility compared with epidemiologic data or local comparison groups. Patients with orofacial injury tended to have high rates of lifetime and current social and mental health needs and were often open in the early recovery phase to considering participation in a positive behavior change program, despite past low levels of social service use.

Given the high rates of unrecognized, untreated psychosocial problems in patients presenting with orofacial injury, using the acute care visits as an opportunity to screen for psychosocial problems will likely increase detection of patients with behavioral disorders and high-risk behaviors that precipitated the injury and that could interfere with a comprehensive recovery. There is evidence that psychosocial screening of trauma patients followed by referral to mental health services for those identified with psychosocial dysfunction may result in improved outcome. Because the acute injury is often the only contact that the patients, who are otherwise healthy young adults, have with the health care system, the hospital encounter provides opportunities to identify problems such as alcohol abuse that would otherwise be missed and lead to subsequent reinjury. Because a significant subset of facial injuries are related to alcohol and substance use,[29] there is potential for incorporating brief screening and behavioral interventions into the care of these patients.

This article has not addressed the often negative psychological and social long-term outcomes of incurring an orofacial injury. As elaborated on in other articles, physical scarring and psychological wounds may develop over time and even become chronic.[10] These negative sequelae can be even more prevalent in persons already experiencing difficulties with substance use, anxiety, depression, hostility, small social networks, limited social support and financial resources, and unmet social service need when they are injured. These results point to the importance of also ascertaining the lifestyle variables associated with sustaining orofacial injuries. Although medical treatment may repair the broken bones, many of these patients continue to be at risk for reinjury or poor psychological outcomes because they may lack the social and personal resources required to sustain any positive behavior changes made. A model of comprehensive intervention built on the principles of collaborative care, wherein practitioners from multiple disciplines work together to develop and implement an integrated treatment plan to address the concurrent social and psychological needs of patients with orofacial injury, seems imperative.[30] In addition to providing surgical care, the team must be able to address social needs (homelessness, joblessness) and psychological needs (PTSD, depression, anxiety, and substance use). Innovative cost-effective programs that can integrate medical and psychological care are especially necessary. Interventions such as motivational interviewing, a brief form of counseling designed to help individuals garner personal resources to promote positive behavior change, which can be offered to patients within days of their facial injury,[31] may be especially important in improving long-term outcomes. However, this collaborative care paradigm requires addressing several clinician, patient, and environmental factors, including attitudinal and procedural barriers to implementing and sustaining psychosocial screening within orofacial injury care: inadequate provider knowledge about mental and behavioral issues and mental health treatment resources in the community, short supply of mental health services and providers, fragmented mental health service systems, and the stigma surrounding mental illness. Training surgeons about behavioral issues, providing easily assessable guides for rapid screening of psychosocial problems, and developing collaborative relationships with mental health professionals and social workers are important first steps toward integrating mental health services into the care of patients with facial injury.

## REFERENCES

1. Bell RB. The role of oral and maxillofacial surgery in the trauma care center. J Oral Maxillofac Surg 2007; 65(12):2544–53.
2. Glynn SM, Asarnow JR, Asarnow R, et al. The development of acute post-traumatic stress disorder after orofacial injury: a prospective study in a large urban hospital. J Oral Maxillofac Surg 2003;61(7):785–92.
3. Bisson JI, Shepherd JP, Joy D, et al. Early cognitive-behavioural therapy for post-traumatic stress symptoms after physical injury: randomised controlled trial. Br J Psychiatry 2004;184:63–9.
4. De Sousa A. Psychological issues in oral and maxillofacial reconstructive surgery. Br J Oral Maxillofac Surg 2008;46(8):661–4.
5. Ogundare BO, Bonnick A, Bayley N. Pattern of mandibular fractures in an urban major trauma center. J Oral Maxillofac Surg 2003;61(6):713–8.
6. Scherer M, Sullivan WG, Smith DJ Jr, et al. An analysis of 1,423 facial fractures in 788 patients at an urban trauma center. J Trauma 1989;29(3):388–90.
7. Auerbach SM, Laskin DM, Kiesler DJ, et al. Psychological factors associated with response to maxillofacial injury and its treatment. J Oral Maxillofac Surg 2008;66(4):755–61.
8. Laski R, Ziccardi VB, Broder HL, et al. Facial trauma: a recurrent disease? The potential role of disease prevention. J Oral Maxillofac Surg 2004;62(6):685–8.
9. Lento J, Glynn S, Shetty V, et al. Psychologic functioning and needs of indigent patients with facial injury: a prospective controlled study. J Oral Maxillofac Surg 2004;62(8):925–32.
10. Glynn SM, Shetty V, Elliot-Brown K, et al. Chronic posttraumatic stress disorder after a facial injury: a 1 year prospective cohort study. J Trauma 2007; 62(2):410–8.
11. Soderstrom CA, Dailey JT, Kerns TJ. Alcohol and other drugs: an assessment of testing and clinical practices in U.S. trauma centers. J Trauma 1994; 36(1):68–73.
12. Babor TF, De La Fuente JR, Saunders J, et al. AUDIT: the alcohol use disorders identification test, guidelines for use in primary health care, in World Health Organization. Geneva, 1989.
13. Wong EC, Marshall GN, Shetty V, et al. Survivors of violence-related facial injury: psychiatric needs and barriers to mental health care. Gen Hosp Psychiatry 2007;29(2):117–22.
14. Cherpitel CJ. A brief screening instrument for problem drinking in the emergency room: the RAPS4. Rapid alcohol problems screen. J Stud Alcohol 2000;61(3):447–9.
15. Zazzali JL, Marshall GN, Shetty V, et al. Provider perceptions of patient psychosocial needs after orofacial injury. J Oral Maxillofac Surg 2007;65(8): 1584–9.
16. Mayfield D, McCleod G, Hall P. The CAGE questionnaire: validation of a new alcoholism screening questionnaire. Am J Psychiatry 1974;131:1121–3.
17. Grant BF, Dawson DA, Stinson FS, et al. The 12-month prevalence and trends in DSM-IV alcohol abuse and dependence: United States, 1991–1992 and 2001–2002. Drug Alcohol Depend 2004;74(3):223–34.
18. Foa EB, Riggs DS, Dancu CV, et al. Reliability and validity of a brief instrument for assessing post-traumatic stress disorder. J Trauma Stress 1993;6:459–73.
19. Breslau N, Kessler RC, Chilcoat HD, et al. Trauma and posttraumatic stress disorder in the community: the 1996 Detroit area survey of trauma. Arch Gen Psychiatry 1998;55(7):626–32.
20. Alim TN, Graves E, Mellman TA, et al. Trauma exposure, posttraumatic stress disorder and depression

in an African-American primary care population. J Natl Med Assoc 2006;98(10):1630–6.

21. Kessler RC, Sonnega A, Bromet E, et al. Posttraumatic stress disorder in the National Comorbidity Survey. Arch Gen Psychiatry 1995;52:1048–60.

22. Asarnow JR, Glynn SM, Asarnow R, et al. Mental health needs of inner-city victims of orofacial injury. Int J Oral Biol 1999;24:31–5.

23. DiClemente CC, Prochaska JO. Toward a comprehensive, transtheoretical model of change: Stages of change and addictive behaviors. In: Miller WR, Heather N, editors. Treating addictive behaviors. 2nd edition. New York: Plenum Press; 1998. p. 3–24.

24. Hall SC, Ofodile FA. Mandibular fractures in an American inner city: the Harlem Hospital Center experience. J Natl Med Assoc 1991;83(5):421–3.

25. Derogatis LR. Brief Symptom Inventory (BSI): administration, scoring, and procedures manual. 3rd edition. Minneapolis (MN): National Computer Systems; 1993.

26. Atchison KA, Gironda MW, Black EE, et al. Baseline characteristics and treatment preferences of oral surgery patients. J Oral Maxillofac Surg 2007; 65(12):2430–7.

27. Piccinelli M, Wilkinson G. Gender differences in depression. Critical review. Br J Psychiatry 2000; 177:486–92.

28. Gater R, Tansella M, Korten A, et al. Sex differences in the prevalence and detection of depressive and anxiety disorders in general health care settings: report from the World Health Organization Collaborative Study on psychological problems in general health care. Arch Gen Psychiatry 1998; 55(5):405–13.

29. Murphy DA, Shetty V, Resell J, et al. Substance use in vulnerable patients with orofacial injury: prevalence, correlates, and unmet service needs. J Trauma 2009;66(2):477–84.

30. Laskin DM. The psychological consequences of maxillofacial injury. J Oral Maxillofac Surg 1999; 57(11):1281.

31. Smith AJ, Hodgson RJ, Bridgeman K, et al. A randomized controlled trial of a brief intervention after alcohol-related facial injury. Addiction 2003; 98(1):43–52.

# The Long-Term Psychological Sequelae of Orofacial Injury

Shirley M. Glynn, PhD[a,b,*], Vivek Shetty, DDS, Dr Med Dent[c]

**KEYWORDS**

• Facial injury • Chronic sequela • Psychosocial • Screening

A growing body of literature has begun to define the variety of psychological difficulties that traumatic injuries can precipitate.[1–4] Common reactions to traumatic events include unwanted reexperiencing of the event, depression, hyperarousal, anxiety, and a persistent sense of current threat. In many instances, the affected individuals are resilient and manifest only short-lived stress reactions that diminish over time without requiring medical or psychological assistance. Nevertheless, in a distinct subset of injured individuals, the constellation of symptoms may be severe enough to meet the diagnostic criteria for posttraumatic stress disorder (PTSD).[5] PTSD is a very debilitating anxiety disorder that can occur after exposure to a terrifying event in which grave physical harm was incurred or threatened.[6,7] Characterized by feelings of fear, helplessness, or horror, the condition is differentiated by the presence of several symptom clusters and elements best summarized by the mnemonic TRAUMA[8]: (1) a Traumatic event occurred in which the person experienced, witnessed, or was confronted by actual or threatened serious injury, death, or threat to the physical integrity of self or other and, as a response to such trauma, the person experienced intense helplessness, fear, and horror; (2) the person Reexperiences such traumatic events through intrusive thoughts, nightmares, flashbacks, or recollection of traumatic memories and images; (3) Avoidance and emotional numbing emerge, expressed as detachment from others; flattening of affect; loss of interest; lack of motivation; and persistent avoidance of activity, places, persons, or events associated with the traumatic experience; (4) symptoms are distressing and cause significant impairment in social, occupational, and interpersonal functioning (patients are Unable to function); (5) these symptoms last for more than 1 Month; (6) the person has increased Arousal, usually manifested by startle reaction, poor concentration, irritable mood, insomnia, and hypervigilance.

Although posttrauma psychopathology can follow any type of trauma exposure, direct exposure such as intentional injury is more likely to be associated with psychiatric sequelae than an indirect exposure to traumatic events.[7] In fact, consensus guidelines from the National Institute of Mental Health identify survivors of violence as a group at high risk for development of PTSD and related comorbid conditions.[9] This recommendation is grounded in the findings of traumatic stress investigators who report the prevalence of chronic PTSD to range from 10% to 30%[3,10] at 12 months postinjury. Through a nationwide study

This work was supported by grant number P50/DE-10598 from the National Institutes of Health/NIDCR.
[a] Research Service, VA Greater Los Angeles Healthcare System at West Los Angeles, B151J, 11301 Wilshire Boulevard, Los Angeles, CA 90073, USA
[b] Semel Institute, University of California, Los Angeles, CA, USA
[c] Section of Oral and Maxillofacial Surgery, 23-009 UCLA School of Dentistry, 10833 Le Conte Avenue, Los Angeles, CA 90095, USA
* Corresponding author. Research Service, VA Greater Los Angeles Healthcare System, West Los Angeles, B151J, 11301 Wilshire Boulevard, Los Angeles, CA 90073.
E-mail address: sglynn@ucla.edu

involving 69 acute care hospitals across the United States, Zatzick and colleagues[4] determined that more than 20% of moderately to severely injured adults had symptoms consistent with a diagnosis of PTSD 12 months after their injury admission. The prevalence of other posttrauma psychopathology is less well known, however, with major depressive episode, generalized anxiety disorder, and substance abuse among the most common comorbid disorders with PTSD. O'Donnell and colleagues[2] found that depression was a common occurrence after injury. The few studies examining comorbid PTSD and depression after injury generally indicate that both disorders frequently co-occur, with between one-half to one-third of injury survivors with PTSD having a comorbid diagnosis of depression.[1,11] The nature of the relationship between PTSD and depression after trauma is complicated. Although both disorders can develop independently after an event, it is also clear that having a previous depressive disorder is a risk factor for the development of subsequent trauma-related PTSD.[12,13] These complex relationships underscore the importance of assessing for both PTSD and depressive symptomatology after traumatic injury.[14]

Persons experiencing intentional orofacial injuries may be particularly vulnerable to the development of chronic PTSD[15] and depression, because these injuries often are intentional[16] and any resultant disfigurement could serve as an ongoing reminder of the event.[17] The development of long-term problems such as chronic PTSD and/or depression in orofacial injury survivors is an area that has only recently begun to attract interest in the clinical research community. In an attempt to clarify long-term psychological sequelae, Sen and colleagues[18] surveyed 1-year psychological outcomes of 147 hospital admissions for orofacial injury. Attrition rates were high (more than 65%), and although the investigators did not formally assess PTSD, they found that 30% of the sample reported persisting high levels of anxiety and depression over the year. This lack of information on the evolution of PTSD and depressive chronicity in orofacial injury survivors has important clinical implications because of the missed opportunities for screening and initiating early psychological interventions to prevent the development or escalation of subsequent mental health problems.

To build a knowledge base on long-term psychological sequelae, this article focuses on the authors' findings relative to posttraumatic psychological outcomes in cohorts of patients with orofacial injury seeking medical care at 2 trauma centers in Los Angeles, the King-Drew Medical Center (KDMC) and the Los Angeles County–University of Southern California Medical Center (LAC-USC). Although the samples differ in important ways (most particularly, participants in the LAC-USC had to have a concurrent substance abuse problem to be eligible for inclusion in the study), distinctive shared characteristics of the 2 samples make them especially informative regarding the prevalence and sequelae of traumatic exposure in this commonly involved, but largely under-studied, vulnerable patient population. These distinctive shared characteristics include gender (predominantly male), ethnicity (predominantly African American and/or Hispanic), limited access to ongoing medical care, and predominance of intentional physical assault as the trauma of interest. In terms of psychological effects, the prospective studies had 3 main goals. First, the authors sought to determine the severity of traumatic stress symptoms in the patient cohorts, 12 months after orofacial injury. Second, in exploratory analyses, they investigated the rates of likely chronic PTSD positive cases 1 year after the injury. Third, they sought to look at the level of depressive symptoms and their trajectory in the LAC-USC sample from which this data was obtained. The authors' overarching objective was to corroborate the findings observed in general trauma settings by determining whether chronic psychopathology was a significant problem in adults recovering from an orofacial injury.

## KDMC STUDY

A study cohort of 336 patients was recruited from the pool of adult patients presenting with orofacial injuries to a level I trauma center in Los Angeles between August 1996 and May 2001.[19,20] Although the spectrum of injury included the mouth, mandible, midfacial, and frontal regions, patients needed to have at least 1 fracture involving the mandible to be eligible for the study. All patients had a similar spectrum of facial injury severity; patients with severe injuries, such as avulsive gunshot injuries, were excluded. Patients with altered mental status attributable to head injuries or who were mentally incompetent were also excluded, as were patients who were unable or unwilling to return for follow-up care. The study procedures were approved by local institutional review boards, and informed consent was obtained from participants.

Concomitant to the surgical treatment, consenting patients were interviewed by research staff using structured questionnaires that included items regarding sociodemographic characteristics and various psychosocial measures. In addition to baseline data collected at the time of admission and discharge, 4 postdischarge patient surveys were administered at the various recall appointments. The first survey was conducted within 10 days of hospital discharge, the second at the 1-month recall appointment, the third approximately 6 months postdischarge, and the fourth approximately 1 year postdischarge.

The Posttraumatic Disorder Scale (PDS)[21] was used to capture lifetime exposure to traumatic events, immediate psychological response, and the subsequent experience of symptoms of PTSD. The PDS was developed specifically as a brief instrument that would help to provide a reliable level of self-reported PTSD symptoms; the structure and content of the PDS mirrors the DSM-IV diagnostic criteria for PTSD.[5] Levels of responses on the scale can be used to suggest a likely diagnosis of PTSD resulting from the injury with high levels of sensitivity and specificity,[22] although subsequent formal diagnostic interviewing is required before a reliable, valid clinical diagnosis can be made. To accommodate the time constraints of a trauma setting, the initial 12 categories of lifetime traumatic exposure were combined into 7 conceptual categories (eg, serious accident, natural disaster, assault [including sexual assault], imprisonment, life-threatening illness, witnessing sudden or violent death, and other life threats).

To establish the levels of traumatic symptoms 1 year after a facial injury and to identify predictors of high rates of chronic PTSD symptoms, the total score on the 12-month PDS was used as the primary dependent measure here; for a secondary analysis, likely positive/negative PTSD diagnostic classifications were made using symptom levels; reports of immediate terror, helplessness, or perceived life threat at the time of the event; and a subsequent decline in role functioning, as specified by Foa.[21] The absolute levels of PDS symptoms at each assessment time point were established. To determine the likely proportion of participants with PTSD from orofacial injury, 12-month PDS responses were scored using the heuristic that was proposed by Foa[21] to classify cases into probable PTSD positive or negative status.

Of the initial study cohort of 336 patients with orofacial injuries, 12-month data were available on 193 participants (57%). Subjects returning for their 12-month follow-ups were predominantly young adult (71% between 18–39 years) ethnic minority (primarily African American and Latinos) males (87.6%). Most of the patients were single (82.4%), unemployed (68.4%), and 33.2% had not graduated from high school. As expected,

PTSD symptoms, manifested by the PDS scores, decreased significantly throughout the year [$F(2, 372) = 10.98$, $P<.001$]; nevertheless, psychological distress scores continued to be high for many individuals. Mean PDS score for the 193 participants at 1 month was 14.14 (standard deviation [SD] 11.97) and at 12 months it was 10.43 (SD 11.31). At the 12-month follow-up, 44 of the returning participants (22.78%) endorsed symptoms consistent with a current PTSD diagnosis on the self-report measure.

With regard to the exposure characteristics of the facial injury, only high levels of pain reported by patients at the 10-day follow-up visit were related to greater severity of PTSD symptoms at 1 month. Prior psychological disturbances, as reflected in lifetime and current mental health needs as well as lifetime social service need and social service use, were the significant predictors of high rates of chronic PTSD symptoms at the 1-year follow-up. Similarly, prior exposure to a traumatic event and high rates of stressful life events in the prior year were strongly predictive of higher PTSD symptoms from the orofacial injury. Perceived social support at the time of the injury was not related to the subsequent development of PTSD; however, a paucity of coping resources in the initial days after the injury, as reflected in not having anyone to count on for instrumental support, not having anyone to count on for emotional support (or needing more emotional support than was available), and having unmet social service needs, was related to higher levels of PTSD symptoms at 12 months. Finally, high scores on the PDS at 1 month were significantly related to high PTSD scores at 12 months.

## LAC-USC STUDY

To extend the findings, the authors conducted similar psychological assessments as part of a randomized controlled trial to test the effectiveness of behavioral interventions addressing antecedent substance use behaviors in patients with orofacial injury. A cohort of 218 patients was recruited from the LAC-USC Medical Center between January 2005 and June 2008. In addition to the criteria used in the KDMC study, eligible patients needed to report regular use of alcohol or illegal drugs in the 6 months before enrollment. After the surgical treatment for their facial injuries, participants were assigned to receive customary care with either motivational interviewing or standard information on substance use behaviors. Similar to the previous study, participants underwent regular assessments, including follow-ups at 6 months and 12 months. To reflect the true longitudinal course of PTSD symptoms in recovery, the authors report the findings only on the educational group.

Psychological responses to the circumstances of the orofacial injury were captured by the PDS, which was described earlier, at the various assessment time points. In addition, the Center for Epidemiologic Studies Depression Scale (CES-D)[23] was used as a measure of depressive symptoms. This 20-item self-test measures depressive feelings and behaviors during the past week and was designed for use in nonclinical settings. Items are scored on a 0 to 3 scale and totaled. The scale has moderate sensitivity and specificity with formal diagnostic interviews of clinical depression.[24] High scores on the CES-D indicate high levels of distress. A score greater than or equal to 16 suggests a clinically significant level of psychological distress.[25] In a general population, about 20% would be expected to score in this range.

Of the initial study cohort of 100 patients with orofacial injury in the education condition, 12-month data on 58 participants (58%) were available. Similar to the previous study, the sample was predominantly young (mean age = 31.1 years), single (60%) males (91%) who were ethnic minorities (74%). The mean PDS score at the time of hospital admission was 16.94 (SD = 13.2). By the 12-month interval, the mean PDS score had dropped to 13.44 (SD = 11.1). The reduction in symptoms over time was marginally significant ($P<.07$); these scores are slightly higher than the sample described earlier. Mean CES-D scores at baseline were 21.4 (SD = 12.7) and 15.54 (SD = 11.8) at 12 months. Although this reduction in depressive symptoms over time was statistically significant ($P<.05$), the overall rates of depressive symptoms endorsed by this sample are still high and close to the cutoff score of 16. These data suggest that many in the sample were experiencing clinical levels of distress that warranted further evaluation. Based on self-report, 42 participants (42%) met the screening criteria for acute PTSD at the 1-month follow-up assessment. At 12-month follow-up, 17 of the returning individuals (30%) reported symptoms on the PDS, suggesting a likely diagnosis of PTSD resulting from the orofacial injury. Of course, formally diagnostic interviewing would be required to make a valid clinical diagnosis.

## GENERALIZABILITY OF THE STUDIES

The authors' studies,[19–20,26–29] among the first to systematically investigate psychological sequelae in patients with facial injury for extended periods of time, have several strengths. Unlike previous limited attempts to clarify postinjury psychopathology, the authors were able to recruit large samples of subjects in public hospital settings. The authors' prospective studies used standardized instruments for repeat assessments conducted over a 1-year period. The sociodemographic characteristics of their subjects, primarily young, single, adult males who were ethnic minorities with limited education and employment, correspond closely to the profiles of patients with facial injury seen at other urban trauma centers. Hence, these features make the authors' investigations particularly informative regarding the psychological needs of high-risk individuals seeking treatment for facial injuries at their urban trauma centers.

The limitations of these studies also merit mention. First, PTSD and depression symptoms and status were rated based on responses to self-report instruments rather than diagnostic interviews. As characteristically happens in services studies that aim to include large patient samples in acute care settings, the authors were forced to weigh the benefits of collecting self-report data from a large sample against the limitations in data interpretation accruing from this method of data collection. Clearly, a replication of the study using interview assessments would be a valuable addition. Nevertheless, the concordance of the self-report versions of the PDS with PTSD diagnosis made using the Structured Clinical Interview for DSM-III-R[22] has been reported to be 79%,[21] with a sensitivity of 82% and a specificity of 76.7%. With regard to the assessment for depression, Boyd and colleagues[24] found, in a community study of 720 subjects, that the sensitivity for major depression as determined by Research Diagnostic Criteria was low (64%) but specificity was high (94%) using a cutoff score of 16. Thus, the authors have some confidence that their results would be replicated with the use of more elaborate interview assessments.

The high number of individuals lost to follow-up is also an issue. To some extent, this attrition likely reflects the transient, limited economic resources in the sample. Many participants were homeless, did not have phones or stable addresses, drifted in and out of prisons or moved around frequently, and were generally difficult to locate for the long-term follow-up interviews. The authors' experiences are not unlike the general difficulty in recruiting and following trauma survivors that is noted by other trauma investigators. Several researchers have suggested that many traumatized individuals use avoidance (eg, refraining from follow-up health care visits) as a primary coping strategy; thus, involvement in a research protocol on long-term psychopathology is in direct contrast to this avoidance and may account for the difficulty in retaining subjects for a period of 1 year. These challenges are illustrated by the study by Roy-Byrne and colleagues[30] who approached 546 emergency room admissions for facial injury to participate in a prospective study on psychological outcomes. Only 56 individuals (10.25%) agreed to participate in their study, and of these, only 32 (57.14%) were available for the 3-month follow-up visit. Although the authors did not have the same difficulties with recruitment, their follow-up numbers reflected a similar difficulty in following people over time, especially for the long-term follow-up assessments.

## IMPLICATIONS FOR CLINICAL PRACTICE

Collectively, the authors' studies begin to illuminate how the experience of orofacial injury can lead to adverse mental health conditions. Although most individuals do recover from the traumatic injury, a significant minority (>20%) will experience high acute stress symptoms that sustain or escalate in the months after the traumatic incident to develop into longer-term psychological disorders. This level of psychopathology is similar to the range noted by O'Donnell and colleagues[3] in their review of general trauma survivors. Although there was a significant reduction in the self-reported depressive symptoms over time, the levels were relatively high both shortly after the traumatic incident and at 12 months postinjury.

As manifest by the traumatic stress literature, injury can disable people in terms of their physical, mental, and/or social functioning.[31,32] Poor mental health seems to be not only one of the most common disabling sequelae of traumatic injury but also the outcome that may hold the most promise for modification by appropriate psychosocial interventions. An individual's own ability to cope with physical impairment, as well as his/her broader social situation, offers opportunities to reduce the extent to which the physical injury can result in disability. By providing people with psychological and social resources that assist their coping responses to the injury, psychosocial interventions may be able to minimize the risk of subsequent orofacial injury resulting in recalcitrant mental, vocational, and social disabilities. The hospital admission for injury management provides a strategic opportunity for identifying individuals who are at risk for adverse psychological sequelae and engaging them with mental health services. Targeted mental health interventions and psychological debriefings during this window of opportunity may prevent the crystallization of abnormal stress reactions into entrenched psychiatric sequelae.

A growing body of literature indicates that individuals with psychopathology such as PTSD may respond to psychotherapeutic and psychopharmacological treatments. For example, the works of Bryant and colleagues[33] and Foa and colleagues[34] have shown that early cognitive behavior therapy interventions delivered in the days and weeks after injury can help to diminish PTSD symptom development. Other investigators such as Hidalgo and Davidson[35] suggest that selective serotonin reuptake inhibitors and tricyclic antidepressants are efficacious treatments for PTSD. Depression is also responsive to treatment, pharmacological[36] and psychological,[37] although relapses are frequent. Similarly, the investigations of Gentillelo and colleagues[38] suggest that motivational interviewing interventions may have utility in decreasing alcohol use in trauma survivors. Taken together, these studies underscore the potential promise of early psychological interventions in the prevention and treatment of posttrauma psychopathology.

Inasmuch as oral and maxillofacial surgeons are typically the primary care providers during the recovery period from an orofacial injury, they are uniquely situated to screen and refer at-risk patients for psychological evaluation and treatment. Assessment of patients with orofacial injury for the risk of developing trauma-related psychopathology can be achieved by simple screenings administered around the time of hospital discharge or during the 1-month follow-up visit when patients return for removal of their maxillomandibular fixation. The 1-month follow-up assessment is particularly useful because many of the transient stress reactions will have diminished by then. Several screening instruments, such as the PDS and CES-D as well as others described in the screening article in this issue, exist that can identify individuals at risk for posttraumatic psychopathology after injury. Sources such as the National Center for PTSD's Web site (http://www.ptsd.va.gov/professional/pages/screening-ptsd-primary-care.asp) are good resources for screening strategies. The total score on these screening measures can be used to classify respondents as being either at "low risk" or "at risk" of developing subsequent psychological sequelae. The process of screening and discussion of mental health and well being during care of the physical injury may also increase the patients' awareness of psychological health and improve their readiness to engage in any necessary mental health interventions. Patients deemed "at risk" can be provided by the surgical team with facilitated referrals to mental health providers in the hospital for follow-up assessments and care.

In summary, significant subsets of patients who experience orofacial injury are at risk for developing psychological sequelae such as PTSD and depression. If undetected and untreated, the psychopathology can become recalcitrant and burden the social and vocational functioning of the patients and greatly diminish their quality of life. The hospital encounter provides the oral and maxillofacial surgeon with opportunities to screen for emerging psychological problems. Several screening instruments are available to assist the surgeon in identifying individuals at risk for subsequent mental health problems. Facilitated referrals to mental health services can be a pragmatic approach for improving comprehensive medical care for these populations and for reducing the potential morbidity of these covert, but disabling, sequelae.

## REFERENCES

1. Shalev AY, Freedman S, Peri T, et al. Prospective study of posttraumatic stress disorder and depression following trauma. Am J Psychiatry 1998; 155(5):630–7. Available at: http://www.ncbi.nlm.nih.gov/pubmed/9585714. Accessed January 5, 2010.
2. O'Donnell ML, Creamer M, Bryant RA, et al. Posttraumatic disorders following injury: an empirical and methodological review. Clin Psychol Rev 2003; 23(4):587–603. Available at: http://www.ncbi.nlm.nih.gov/pubmed/12788111. Accessed January 5, 2010.
3. O'Donnell ML, Creamer M, Pattison P, et al. Psychiatric morbidity following injury. Am J Psychiatry 2004;161(3):507–14. Available at: http://www.ncbi.nlm.nih.gov/pubmed/14992977. Accessed January 5, 2010.
4. Zatzick DF, Rivara FP, Nathens AB, et al. A nationwide US study of post-traumatic stress after hospitalization for physical injury. Psychol Med 2007; 37(10):1469–80. Available at: http://www.ncbi.nlm.nih.gov/pubmed/17559704. Accessed January 5, 2010.
5. American Psychiatric Association. Diagnostic and Statistical Manual of Mental Disorders (DSM-IV). Washington, DC: American Psychiatric Association; 1994.
6. Shalev AY. Posttraumatic stress disorder and stress-related disorders. Psychiatr Clin North Am 2009; 32(3):687–704. Available at: http://www.ncbi.nlm.nih.gov/pubmed/19716997. Accessed January 5, 2010.
7. Yehuda R. Post-traumatic stress disorder. N Engl J Med 2002;346(2):108–14. Available at: http://content.nejm.org. Accessed January 5, 2010.
8. Khouzam HR. A simple mnemonic for the diagnostic criteria for post-traumatic stress disorder. West J Med 2001;174(6):424. Available at: http://www.ncbi.nlm.nih.gov/pubmed/11381013. Accessed January 5, 2010.
9. National Institute of Mental Health. Mental health and mass violence: evidence-based early psychological intervention for victims/survivors of mass violence. A workshop to reach consensus on best practices. (2002). NIH Publication No. 02-5138. National Institute of Mental Health: Washington, DC;2002.
10. Zatzick DF, Jurkovich GJ, Gentilello L, et al. Posttraumatic stress, problem drinking, and functional outcomes after injury. Arch Surg 2002; 137(2):200–5. Available at: http://www.ncbi.nlm.nih.gov/pubmed/11822960. Accessed January 5, 2010.
11. Blanchard EB, Hickling EJ, Galovski T, et al. Emergency room vital signs and PTSD in a treatment seeking sample of motor vehicle accident survivors. J Trauma Stress 2002;15(3):199–204. Available at: http://www.ncbi.nlm.nih.gov/pubmed/12092911. Accessed January 5, 2010.
12. Acierno R, Resnick H, Kilpatrick DG, et al. Risk factors for rape, physical assault, and posttraumatic stress disorder in women: examination of differential multivariate relationships. J Anxiety Disord 1999; 13(6):541–63. Available at: http://www.ncbi.nlm.nih.gov/pubmed/10688523. Accessed January 10, 2010.
13. Resnick HS, Kilpatrick DG, Best CL, et al. Vulnerability-stress factors in development of posttraumatic stress disorder. J Nerv Ment Dis 1992;180(7):424–30. Available at: http://www.ncbi.nlm.nih.gov/pubmed/1624923. Accessed January 10, 2010.
14. Brady KT, Killeen TK, Brewerton T, et al. Comorbidity of psychiatric disorders and posttraumatic stress disorder. J Clin Psychiatry 2000;61(Suppl 7):22–32. Available at: http://www.ncbi.nlm.nih.gov/pubmed/10795606. Accessed January 5, 2010.
15. Hull AM, Lowe T, Finlay PM. The psychological impact of maxillofacial trauma: an overview of reactions to trauma. Oral Surg Oral Med Oral Pathol Oral Radiol Endod 2003;95(5):515–20. Available at: http://www.ncbi.nlm.nih.gov/pubmed/12738941. Accessed January 5, 2010.
16. Scherer M, Sullivan WG, Smith DJ, et al. An analysis of 1,423 facial fractures in 788 patients at an urban trauma center. J Trauma 1989;29(3):388–90. Available at: http://www.ncbi.nlm.nih.gov/pubmed/2648018. Accessed January 5, 2010.
17. Thompson A, Kent G. Adjusting to disfigurement: processes involved in dealing with being visibly different. Clin Psychol Rev 2001;21(5):663–82.

Available at: http://www.ncbi.nlm.nih.gov/pubmed/ 11434225. Accessed January 5, 2010.

18. Sen P, Ross N, Rogers S. Recovering maxillofacial trauma patients: the hidden problems. J Wound Care 2001;10(3):53–7. Available at: http://www.ncbi. nlm.nih.gov/pubmed/11924351. Accessed January 5, 2010.

19. Glynn SM, Shetty V, Elliot-Brown K, et al. Chronic post-traumatic stress disorder after facial injury: a 1-year prospective cohort study. J Trauma 2007;62(2): 410–8 [discussion: 418]. Available at: http://www. ncbi.nlm.nih.gov/pubmed/17297333. Accessed August 31, 2009.

20. Glynn SM, Asarnow JR, Asarnow R, et al. The development of acute post-traumatic stress disorder after orofacial injury: a prospective study in a large urban hospital. J Oral Maxillofac Surg 2003;61(7):785–92. Available at: http://www.ncbi.nlm.nih.gov/pubmed/ 12856251. Accessed August 31, 2009.

21. Foa E, Cashman L, Jaycox L, et al. The validation of a self-report measure of posttraumatic stress disorder: the posttraumatic diagnostic scale. Psychol Assess 1977;9:445–51.

22. Spitzer RL, Williams JB, Gibbon M, et al. The structured clinical interview for DSM-III-R (SCID). I: history, rationale, and description. Arch Gen Psychiatry 1992;49(8):624–9. Available at: http://www.ncbi. nlm.nih.gov/pubmed/1637252. Accessed January 6, 2010.

23. Radloff L. The CES-D Scale: a Self-Report Depression Scale for research in the general population. Appl Psychol Meas 1977;1:385–401.

24. Boyd JH, Weissman MM, Thompson WD, et al. Screening for depression in a community sample. Understanding the discrepancies between depression symptom and diagnostic scales. Arch Gen Psychiatry 1982;39(10):1195–200. Available at: http://www.ncbi.nlm.nih.gov/pubmed/7125849. Accessed January 6, 2010.

25. Weissman MM, Sholomskas D, Pottenger M, et al. Assessing depressive symptoms in five psychiatric populations: a validation study. Am J Epidemiol 1977;106(3):203–14. Available at: http://www.ncbi. nlm.nih.gov/pubmed/900119. Accessed January 6, 2010.

26. Lento J, Glynn S, Shetty V, et al. Psychologic functioning and needs of indigent patients with facial injury: a prospective controlled study. J Oral Maxillofac Surg 2004;62(8):925–32. Available at: http://www.ncbi.nlm.nih.gov/pubmed/15278855. Accessed July 26, 2008.

27. Lui A, Glynn S, Shetty V. The interplay of perceived social support and posttraumatic psychological distress following orofacial injury. J Nerv Ment Dis 2009;197(9):639–45. Available at: http://journals. lww.com/jonmd/pages/articleviewer.aspx?year=

2009&issue=09000&article=00001&type=abstract. Accessed October 22, 2009.

28. Marshall GN, Schell TL, Glynn SM, et al. The role of hyperarousal in the manifestation of posttraumatic psychological distress following injury. J Abnorm Psychol 2006;115(3):624–8. Available at: http://www.ncbi.nlm.nih.gov/pubmed/16866603. Accessed August 27, 2008.

29. Shetty V, Dent DM, Glynn S, et al. Psychosocial sequelae and correlates of orofacial injury. Dent Clin North Am 2003;47(1):141–57, xi. Available at: http://www.ncbi.nlm.nih.gov/pubmed/12519011. Accessed July 26, 2008.

30. Roy-Byrne PP, Russo J, Michelson E, et al. Risk factors and outcome in ambulatory assault victims presenting to the acute emergency department setting: implications for secondary prevention studies in PTSD. Depress Anxiety 2004;19(2): 77–84. Available at: http://www.ncbi.nlm.nih.gov/ pubmed/15022142. Accessed January 6, 2010.

31. McFarlane AC. Posttraumatic stress disorder: a model of the longitudinal course and the role of risk factors. J Clin Psychiatry 2000;61(Suppl 5):15–20 [discussion: 21–3]. Available at: http://www.ncbi.nlm.nih.gov/ pubmed/10761675. Accessed January 6, 2010.

32. Kulka RA, Schlenger WE, Fairbank JA, et al. Trauma and the Vietnam war generation: report of the findings from the national Vietnam veterans readjustment study. New York: Brunner/Mazel; 1990.

33. Bryant RA, Harvey AG, Dang ST, et al. Treatment of acute stress disorder: a comparison of cognitive-behavioral therapy and supportive counseling. J Consult Clin Psychol 1998;66(5):862–6. Available at: http://www.ncbi.nlm.nih.gov/pubmed/9803707. Accessed January 6, 2010.

34. Foa EB, Hearst-Ikeda D, Perry KJ. Evaluation of a brief cognitive-behavioral program for the prevention of chronic PTSD in recent assault victims. J Consult Clin Psychol 1995;63(6):948–55. Available at: http://www.ncbi.nlm.nih.gov/pubmed/8543717. Accessed January 6, 2010.

35. Hidalgo RB, Davidson JR. Selective serotonin reuptake inhibitors in post-traumatic stress disorder. J Psychopharmacol 2000;14(1):70–6. Available at: http://www.ncbi.nlm.nih.gov/pubmed/10757257. Accessed January 6, 2010.

36. Pampallona S, Bollini P, Tibaldi G, et al. Combined pharmacotherapy and psychological treatment for depression: a systematic review. Arch Gen Psychiatry 2004;61(7):714–9. Available at: http://www. ncbi.nlm.nih.gov/pubmed/15237083. Accessed January 6, 2010.

37. Lau MA. New developments in psychosocial interventions for adults with unipolar depression. Curr Opin Psychiatry 2008;21(1):30–6. Available

at: http://www.ncbi.nlm.nih.gov/pubmed/18281838. Accessed January 6, 2010.

38. Gentilello LM, Rivara FP, Donovan DM, et al. Alcohol interventions in a trauma center as a means of reducing the risk of injury recurrence. Ann Surg 1999;230(4):473–80 [discussion: 480–3]. Available at: http://www.ncbi.nlm.nih.gov/pubmed/10522717. Accessed January 6, 2010.

# Screening for Psychiatric Problems in the Orofacial Trauma Setting

Grant N. Marshall, PhD

**KEYWORDS**

• Orofacial trauma • PTSD • Depressive disorder

Persons who sustain orofacial trauma not only require restoration of physical anatomy and functional status but also may have a need for trauma-related mental services. In particular, survivors of orofacial trauma are at an elevated risk of posttraumatic stress disorder (PTSD)[1–4] as well as major depressive disorder.[4–6] Fortunately, efficacious treatments for both conditions are available.[7–11] Given the frequency with which PTSD and major depression may develop in facial injury survivors, frontline providers of services to patients with orofacial trauma must be able to recognize and screen for these psychiatric disorders.

## WHAT IS PTSD?

PTSD is a psychiatric disorder that may follow exposure to a traumatic life event. An event is regarded as traumatic if it involves either actual or threatened death or serious injury. To qualify as traumatic, the event must also trigger intense fear, helplessness, or horror during or immediately after it takes place. PTSD is characterized by 3 clusters of symptoms: (1) persistent and intrusive distressing recollections of the event (eg, nightmares, flashbacks), (2) avoidance of reminders of the event (eg, efforts to avoid thoughts or places associated with the trauma) or numbing of general responsiveness (eg, a manifest loss of interest in previously pleasurable activities), and (3) persistent symptoms of hyperarousal (eg, hypervigilance, difficulty falling asleep).[12] Symptoms must

last for more than 1 month and cause either clinically significant distress or impairment in functioning to meet diagnostic criteria for PTSD. Many individuals experience transient psychological distress in the immediate aftermath of trauma exposure. This distress is typically self-limited, with spontaneous recovery occurring within several days or a few weeks. Thus, PTSD can be distinguished from more transient reactions to stress by reference to symptom duration.

## HOW COMMON IS PTSD?

PTSD is a relatively common psychiatric condition, with a lifetime prevalence of approximately 8% in the general population.[13,14] The disorder occurs frequently in trauma settings, with studies suggesting an incidence of approximately 20% in the months immediately after hospitalization for the treatment of traumatic physical injury.[15,16]

## SCREENING FOR PTSD

Although a definitive diagnosis of PTSD requires a clinical interview, screening tools exist to assist orofacial trauma care providers in identifying patients who might benefit from referral for a more detailed mental health evaluation. Various screening instruments have been developed that assess the severity and/or frequency of symptoms of PTSD as found in the Diagnostic and Statistical Manual of Mental Disorders, fourth edition (DSM-IV) (for a review, see Brewin's article[17]). Among

Preparation of this manuscript was supported by grant number R34MH071569 from the National Institute of Mental Health.
RAND Corporation, 1776 Main Street, Santa Monica, CA 90407, USA
E-mail address: grantm@rand.org

the most commonly used instruments are the PTSD Symptom Checklist,[18] the Posttraumatic Diagnostic Scale,[19] the revised version of the Impact of Event Scale,[20] and the Davidson Trauma Scale.[21] For example, the PTSD Symptom Checklist assesses for the presence of all 17 symptoms of PTSD. Items are phrased in the form of statements, and respondents indicate the extent to which they have been bothered by each symptom in the past week.[18]

Although completion of these screeners is substantially less burdensome than administration of a diagnostic interview, each screener contains a minimum of 17 items corresponding to the 17 symptoms of PTSD. Thus, even these brief tools may be insufficiently short for use in busy clinical care settings. To satisfy the need for a concise screening tool to identify patients with possible PTSD, several short screeners have been developed. One such screener, the 4-item Startle, Physiologic arousal, Anger, and Numbness (SPAN) instrument[22] was derived from the Davidson Trauma Scale. To complete the SPAN, respondents are asked to identify the trauma that was most disturbing and to assess the degree to which each of the 4 symptoms has distressed them during the past week. The symptoms that compose the SPAN are those that best distinguish a sample of patients with PTSD from a comparison sample of persons without PTSD (responses are provided with respect to a 5-point scale ranging from 0 = "not at all" to 4 = "extremely distressing"). Scores of 5 or more indicate possible PTSD.

The SPAN was initially validated using a sample of 243 persons exposed to various types of trauma (eg, combat, natural disaster) who had been diagnosed with PTSD via a clinical interview.[22] In the validation sample, the SPAN had a sensitivity of 0.84 (ie, the proportion of all positive cases that were detected) and a specificity of 0.91 (ie, the proportion of all negative cases that were detected) in the original sample of heterogeneous trauma survivors. In a subsequent validation subsample, a cut score of 5 or more points resulted in a sensitivity of 0.77 and a specificity of 0.82. Further research attests to the utility of the SPAN as a brief PTSD screener in various traumatized populations.[23,24]

A second short PTSD screening tool was adapted from an instrument originally developed to screen for lifetime PTSD in community samples.[25] As adapted by Kimerling and colleagues,[26,27] this screener consists of 7 PTSD symptoms, with respondents indicating whether or not each symptom had been experienced in the preceding month. The screener was validated using a sample of 134 medical outpatients. A cut point of 4 or

more symptoms had a sensitivity of 0.85 and a specificity of 0.84 for identifying persons with PTSD in a primary care setting.

A third PTSD screener, the Primary Care PTSD (PC-PTSD), was developed expressly for use in primary care.[28] Consisting of items assessing 4 PTSD symptoms, this instrument was initially developed using data from 188 patients in primary care. To complete the screener, respondents indicate whether they have experienced each symptom in the past month. Endorsement of 3 or more symptoms of the PC-PTSD is suggestive of PTSD. A cut point greater than or equal to 3 has a sensitivity of 0.78 and a specificity of 0.87, relative to a structured diagnostic interview. Subsequent research has shown that the PC-PTSD performs well as a screener in various settings.[26,29,30]

The SPAN, the instrument developed by Kimerling and colleagues,[26,27] and the PC-PTSD can be administered as a brief interview. Moreover, each is suitable for self-administration for most patients. As determined by the Flesch-Kincaid grade level readability test,[31] the SPAN is capable of being read by individuals with a sixth grade education, whereas the PC-PTSD requires an eighth grade reading level. Self-administration of the screener developed by Kimerling and colleagues[26,27] requires an estimated 10th grade reading level. Thus, the latter screener is perhaps less useful than the others as a self-administered tool.

## PTSD SUMMARY

PTSD is common in survivors of orofacial trauma. Although definitive determination of the presence of PTSD requires a time-intensive diagnostic interview, brief and easily administered screening instruments can aid in the identification of patients who may benefit from referral for further evaluation and possible treatment. Given that PTSD requires the presence of symptoms for a period of at least 30 days, a 1-month follow-up wound check visit would be an ideal time to screen for the presence of PTSD. The SPAN,[22] Kimerling and colleagues' instrument,[26,27] and the PC-PTSD[28] all possess desirable features as screening tools. The evidence attesting to the utility of these instruments is good, although additional research is needed. In particular, no studies have examined the validity of these PTSD screeners against diagnostic interviews in the trauma center context.

## WHAT IS MAJOR DEPRESSION?

Major depressive disorder is a psychiatric condition anchored by depressed mood and loss of interest or pleasure. At least 5 of the following symptoms must have been present for a 2-week period accompanied by either depressed mood or loss of interest: depressed mood, loss of interest or pleasure, appetite disturbance, sleep disturbance, psychomotor agitation or retardation, fatigue, feelings of worthlessness or excessive guilt, difficulty concentrating, and recurrent thoughts of death.[12] Symptoms must cause either clinically significant distress or impairment in functioning to meet diagnostic criteria for major depression.

## HOW COMMON IS MAJOR DEPRESSION?

Major depressive disorder is widespread in the general population, with a lifetime prevalence of nearly 17%.[14] The disorder is increasingly recognized as common in the aftermath of physical trauma.[32–34] For example, in a study of 212 patients with general trauma, Shalev and colleagues[34] reported that 19% met DSM-IV diagnostic criteria for major depression at 1 month postinjury, whereas 14% were diagnosable at 4 months posttrauma.[34]

## SCREENING FOR MAJOR DEPRESSION

Numerous screening instruments have been developed to assess for major depression. Some of the most widely known instruments include the Center for Epidemiologic Studies Depression Scale,[35] the Zung Self-Rating Depression Scale,[36] and the Beck Depression Inventory.[37,38] For example, the Zung Depression Scale consists of 20 symptoms phrased as statements (eg, I feel downhearted and blue), with respondents indicating the extent to which each symptom has been experienced in the past several days. Responses are provided on a 4-point scale ranging from "a little of the time" to "most of the time."[36]

Because even these short depression screeners often contain 20 or more items, administration in busy treatment settings can be burdensome for staff and respondents. For this reason, considerable attention has been devoted to the development of even shorter depression screener tools for use in clinical contexts. The Patient Health Questionnaire (PHQ-9) has attracted considerable attention as a depression screener.[39] This instrument was developed for use in primary care settings and consists of 9 items. Phrased as statements, each item is answered with respect to the past 2 weeks. Respondents indicate the extent to which each symptom bothered them on a 4-point scale, with response options consisting of 0 = not at all, 1 = several days, 2 = more than half the days,

and 3 = nearly every day. Major depression is suggested if respondents endorse 5 or more of the 9 symptoms as having been present more than half of the days in the past 2 weeks. A more lenient threshold may also be used as an indicator of a milder episode of depression. In either instance, individuals who receive screening scores exceeding the relevant cut point may benefit from referral for further evaluation.

In the original validation research conducted with approximately 6000 patients in 8 primary care and 7 obstetrics/gynecology clinics, the PHQ-9 was found to have a sensitivity of 0.88 and a specificity of 0.88 for major depressive disorder.[39] Subsequent investigations of the PHQ-9 have demonstrated that the instrument possesses utility as a depression screener in various contexts and settings.[40–48] For example, in a sample of 440 primary care patients, Wittkampf and colleagues[48] reported that the PHQ-9 performed well as a screener for major depression as assessed by a structured clinical interview.

A small but growing body of research suggests that a 2-item version of the PHQ-9 might also perform well as a screener for depression in various settings.[49–53] Although a 2-item scale has considerable practical appeal, some evidence suggests that this tool may result in too many "false positive" screens. In particular, Gjerdingen and colleagues[49] reported a sensitivity of 100% but a specificity of only 44% in their study of postpartum depression. These investigators have recommended that the PHQ-2 might be administered as part of a 2-phase process in which individuals who screen positive on the 2-item screener are then administered the full PHQ-9. Other research has indicated, however, that the 2-phase approach to using the PHQ-9 may not be superior to using either the PHQ-2 or the PHQ-9 by itself.[54] The potential for "false positive" screens in the context of orofacial trauma would more than offset the reduction in administrative burden associated with the use of the PHQ-2. Although additional research may ultimately support the utility of the PHQ-2 for use in the orofacial trauma setting, in the absence of this evidence, it may be premature to rely solely on the PHQ-2 in screening for depression in this context.

The PHQ-9 is intended for self-administration, and the instrument is readable by persons with a seventh grade education as determined by the Flesch-Kincaid grade level readability test.[31]

## DEPRESSION SUMMARY

Major depressive disorder is common in survivors of orofacial trauma. Although a complete diagnostic interview is required to make a definitive diagnosis of major depression, brief screening instruments are available to assist in identifying patients who may benefit from referral for mental health evaluation. Of these instruments, the PHQ-9 is rapidly becoming the most widely used depression screener. Evidence attests to the validity of the PHQ-9, although additional research is needed to assess its validity for use as a screener in the orofacial trauma context.

## REFERENCES

1. Bisson JI, Shepherd JP, Dhutia M. Psychological sequelae of facial trauma. J Trauma 1997;43: 496–500.
2. Glynn SM, Asarnow JR, Asarnow R, et al. The development of acute post-traumatic stress disorder after orofacial injury: a prospective study in a large urban hospital. J Oral Maxillofac Surg 2003;61:785–92.
3. Lento J, Glynn S, Shetty V, et al. Psychologic functioning and needs of indigent patients with facial injury: a prospective controlled study. J Oral Maxillofac Surg 2004;62:925–32.
4. Roccia F, Dell'Acqua A, Angelini G, et al. Maxillofacial trauma and psychiatric sequelae: post-traumatic stress disorder. J Craniofac Surg 2005;16: 355–60.
5. Gironda MW, Der-Martirosian C, Belin TR, et al. Predictors of depressive symptoms following mandibular fracture repair. Oral Maxillofac Surg 2009;67:328–34.
6. Hull AM, Lowe T, Devlin M, et al. Psychological consequences of maxillofacial trauma: a preliminary study. Br J Oral Maxillofac Surg 2003;41:317–22.
7. Anderson IM, Ferrier IN, Baldwin RC, et al. Evidence-based guidelines for treating depressive disorders with antidepressants: a revision of the 2000 British Association for Psychopharmacology guidelines. J Psychopharmacol 2008;22:343–96.
8. Foa EB, Friedman MJ, Keane TM. Effective treatments for PTSD: practice guidelines from the International Society for Traumatic Stress Studies. New York: Guildford; 2004.
9. Kuyken W, Dalgleish T, Holden ER. Advances in cognitive-behavioural therapy for unipolar depression. Can J Psychiatry 2007;52:5–13.
10. Malhi GS, Adams D, Porter R, et al. Clinical practice recommendations for depression. Acta Psychiatr Scand 2009;119(Suppl 439):8–26.
11. Stein DJ, Ipser JC, Seedat S. Pharmacotherapy for post traumatic stress disorder (PTSD). Cochrane Database Syst Rev 2006;(1):CD002795.
12. American Psychiatric Association. Diagnostic and statistical manual of mental disorders. 4th edition. Washington, DC: Author; 1994.
13. Kessler RC, Sonnega A, Bromet E, et al. Posttraumatic stress disorder in the National Comorbidity Survey. Arch Gen Psychiatry 1995;52:1048–60.
14. Kessler RC, Berglund P, Demler O, et al. Lifetime prevalence and age-of-onset distributions of DSM-IV disorders in the National Comorbidity Survey Replication. Arch Gen Psychiatry 2005;62:593–602.
15. Marshall GN, Miles JN, Stewart SH. Anxiety sensitivity and PTSD symptom severity are reciprocally related: evidence from a longitudinal study of physical trauma survivors. J Abnorm Psychol 2010; 119(1):143–50.
16. Zatzick DF, Rivara FP, Nathens AB, et al. A nationwide US study of post-traumatic stress after hospitalization for physical injury. Psychol Med 2007;37: 1469–80.
17. Brewin CR. Systematic review of screening instruments for adults at risk of PTSD. J Trauma Stress 2005;18:53–62.
18. Weathers FW, Litz BT, Herman DS, et al. The PTSD Checklist (PCL): reliability, validity, and diagnostic utility. Ninth Annual Meeting of the International Society for Traumatic Stress Studies. San Antonio, TX. 1993. Available at: http://www.pdhealth.mil/library/downloads/PCL_sychometrics.doc. Accessed December 1, 2009.
19. Foa EB, Cashman L, Jaycox L, et al. The validation of a self-report measure of posttraumatic stress disorder: the Posttraumatic Diagnostic Scale. Psychol Assess 1997;9:445–51.
20. Weiss DS, Marmar CR. The Impact of Event Scale—revised. In: Wilson JP, Keane TM, editors. Assessing psychological trauma and PTSD. New York: Guilford Press; 1997. p. 399–411.
21. Davidson JRT, Book SW, Colket JT, et al. Assessment of a new self-rating scale for post-traumatic stress disorder. Psychol Med 1997;27:153–60.
22. Meltzer-Brody S, Churchill E, Davidson JR. Derivation of the SPAN, a brief diagnostic screening test for posttraumatic stress disorder. Psychiatry Res 1999;88:63–70.
23. Meltzer-Brody S, Hartmann K, Miller WC, et al. A brief screening instrument to detect posttraumatic stress disorder in outpatient gynecology. Obstet Gynecol 2004;104:770–6.
24. Yeager DE, Magruder KM, Knapp RG, et al. Performance characteristics of the Posttraumatic Stress Disorder Checklist and SPAN in Veterans Affairs primary care settings. Gen Hosp Psychiatry 2007; 29:294–301.
25. Breslau N, Peterson EL, Kessler RC, et al. Short screening scale for DSM-IV posttraumatic stress disorder. Am J Psychiatry 1999;156:908–11.
26. Kimerling R, Trafton JA, Nguyen B. Validation of a brief screen for post-traumatic stress disorder with substance use disorder patients. Addict Behav 2006;31:2074–9.

27. Kimerling R, Ouimette P, Prins A, et al. Utility of a short screening scale for DSM-IV PTSD in primary care. J Gen Intern Med 2006;21:65–7.

28. Prins A, Ouimet P, Kimerling R, et al. The primary care PTSD screen (PC-PTSD): development and operating characteristics. Prim Care Psychiatr 2004;9:9–14.

29. Bliese PD, Wright KM, Adler AB, et al. Validating the primary care posttraumatic stress disorder screen and the posttraumatic stress disorder checklist with soldiers returning from combat. J Consult Clin Psychol 2008;76:272–81.

30. Reger MA, Gahm GA, Swanson RD, et al. Association between number of deployments to Iraq and mental health screening outcomes in US army soldiers. J Clin Psychiatry 2009;70:1266–72.

31. Kincaid JP, Fishburne RP Jr, Rogers RL, et al. Derivation of new readability formulas (Automated Readability Index, Fog Count and Flesch Reading Ease Formula) for Navy enlisted personnel, Research Branch Report 8-75. Millington (TN): Naval Technical Training; 1975. Memphis (TN): U.S. Naval Air Station.

32. Blanchard EB, Buckley TC, Hickling EJ, et al. Posttraumatic stress disorder and comorbid major depression: is the correlation an illusion? J Anxiety Disord 1998;12:21–37.

33. Islam S, Ahmed M, Walton GM, et al. The association between depression and anxiety disorders following facial trauma—a comparative study. Injury 2010;41(1):92–6.

34. Shalev AY, Freedman S, Peri T, et al. Prospective study of posttraumatic stress disorder and depression following trauma. Am J Psychiatry 1998;155:630–7.

35. Radloff LS. The CES-D Scale: a self-report depression scale for research in the general population. Appl Psychol Meas 1977;1:385–401.

36. Zung WW. A self-rating depression scale. Arch Gen Psychiatry 1965;12:63–70.

37. Beck AT, Ward CH, Mendelson M, et al. An inventory for measuring depression. Arch Gen Psychiatry 1961;4:561–71.

38. Beck AT, Steer RA, Ball R, et al. Comparison of Beck depression Inventories -IA and -II in psychiatric outpatients. J Pers Assess 1996;67:588–97.

39. Kroenke K, Spitzer RL, Williams JB. The PHQ-9: validity of a brief depression severity measure. J Gen Intern Med 2001;16:606–13.

40. Bombardier CH, Richards JS, Krause JS, et al. Symptoms of major depression in people with spinal cord injury: implications for screening. Arch Phys Med Rehabil 2004;85:1749–56.

41. Chen TM, Huang FY, Chang C, et al. Using the PHQ-9 for depression screening and treatment monitoring for Chinese Americans in primary care. Psychiatr Serv 2006;57:976–81.

42. Fann JR, Bombardier CH, Dikmen S, et al. Validity of the Patient Health Questionnaire-9 in assessing depression following traumatic brain injury. J Head Trauma Rehabil 2005;20:501–11.

43. Hansson M, Chotai J, Nordstöm A, et al. Comparison of two self-rating scales to detect depression: HADS and PHQ-9. Br J Gen Pract 2009;59:283–8.

44. Martin A, Rief W, Klaiberg A, et al. Validity of the Brief Patient Health Questionnaire Mood Scale (PHQ-9) in the general population. Gen Hosp Psychiatry 2006;28:71–7.

45. Pinto-Meza A, Serrano-Blanco A, Peñarrubia MT, et al. Assessing depression in primary care with the PHQ-9: can it be carried out over the telephone? J Gen Intern Med 2005;20:738–42.

46. Reuland DS, Cherrington A, Watkins GS, et al. Diagnostic accuracy of Spanish language depression-screening instruments. J Trauma Stress 2009;7:455–62.

47. Williams LS, Brizendine EJ, Plue L, et al. Performance of the PHQ-9 as a screening tool for depression after stroke. Stroke 2005;36:635–8.

48. Wittkampf K, van Ravesteijn H, Baas K, et al. The accuracy of Patient Health Questionnaire-9 in detecting depression and measuring depression severity in high-risk groups in primary care. Gen Hosp Psychiatry 2009;31:451–9.

49. Gjerdingen D, Crow S, McGovern P, et al. Postpartum depression screening at well-child visits: validity of a 2-question screen and the PHQ-9. Ann Fam Med 2009;7:63–70.

50. Kroenke K, Spritzer RL, Williams JBW. The Patient Health Questionnaire-2: validity of a two-item depression screener. Med Care 2003;41:1284–92.

51. Löwe B, Kroenke K, Gräfe K. Detecting and monitoring depression with a two-item questionnaire (PHQ-2). J Psychosom Res 2005;58:163–71.

52. Mitchell AJ, McGlinchey JB, Young D, et al. Accuracy of specific symptoms in the diagnosis of major depressive disorder in psychiatric out-patients: data from the MIDAS project. Psychol Med 2009;39:1107–16.

53. Watson LC, Zimmerman S, Cohen LW, et al. Practical depression screening in residential care/assisted living: five methods compared with gold standard diagnoses. Am J Geriatr Psychiatry 2009;17:556–64.

54. Thombs BD, Ziegelstein RC, Whooley MA. Optimizing detection of major depression among patients with coronary artery disease using the patient health questionnaire: data from the heart and soul study. J Gen Intern Med 2008;23:2014–7.

# Substance Use and Facial Injury

Debra A. Murphy, PhD

**KEYWORDS**

- Substance use • Facial injury • Trauma centers

The use of alcohol and illicit drugs is a common theme in patients presenting with traumatic injury to trauma centers. In addition to associated patient care issues, these common precipitants of clinician contact and costly hospitalizations present a particular fiscal challenge to our trauma care systems and compromise their ability to provide conventional medical services. Estimates compiled by the Institute of Medicine's Committee on Injury Prevention and Control indicate that the costs of injury are higher than those of any other health problem, and are roughly equal to the costs associated with heart disease (second most costly) and cancer (third most costly) combined.[1] Similar injury trends are increasingly manifest in children and adolescents[2,3]; between 2002 and 2004, more than 13 million emergency department visits in the United States involved adolescents 10 to 19 years of age, with injury constituting 42% of these visits.[4] Given that alcohol and substance use are common antecedent risk factors for traumatic injury, a significant portion of facial injuries should be considered as preventable.

The focus of this article is to: (1) detail the connection between substance use and orofacial injuries among adults and adolescents, (2) discuss the sequelae of substance-use–related orofacial injuries (ie, complications and reinjury), and (3) discuss the need for collaborative care across disciplines.

## SUBSTANCE USE AND INJURY AMONG ADULTS

A sizable proportion of adults receiving treatment at trauma centers exhibit a pattern of harmful substance-using behaviors. For example, pooled data on 4063 patients treated at 6 regional trauma centers indicated that 40.2% of patients had a positive blood alcohol concentration at admission[5]; when polydrug use (alcohol, illicit drugs) was included, more than 60% of patients tested positive for intoxicants.[6] These findings reflect the results of Cornwell and colleagues,[7] who investigated the prevalence of substance use among victims of major trauma presenting to a level I trauma center. Of the 516 patients who had urine toxicology and blood alcohol screens, 71% screened positive for alcohol or drugs, or both; 52% had positive alcohol screens; and 42% had positive drug screens with cocaine and opiates representing 91% of positive drug screens.

As with general trauma, there are substantive linkages between substance use and facial injury. Mathog and colleagues[8] found that more than 82% of the 1432 mandible fractures in 906 patients were the result of aggravated assault and were related largely to substance use and risky behaviors. Their findings are echoed by Ogundare and colleagues,[9] who reported interpersonal violence as the proximate cause of injury in 79% of all patients with mandible fractures, with 55% of the patients reporting the use of an illicit substance within 2 hours of the injury. Murphy and colleagues[10] found that 58% of patients presenting with intentional facial injury at an urban trauma center met criteria for problem drinking, and over half reported illicit substance use in the previous month, with 25% meeting criteria for problem drug use. Similarly, the association of alcohol use with interpersonal violence was 72% in an audit of emergency referrals to a maxillofacial trauma unit over a period of 2 years.[11]

This work was supported by Grants Nos. 5R21DE016490 and 5R01DA016850 from the National Institutes of Health.

Health Risk Reduction Projects, Integrated Substance Abuse Programs, Department of Psychiatry, University of California, 11075 Santa Monica Boulevard, Suite 200, Los Angeles, CA 90025-7539, USA

E-mail address: dmurphy@mednet.ucla.edu

Oral Maxillofacial Surg Clin N Am 22 (2010) 231–238
doi:10.1016/j.coms.2010.01.005

Most studies conducted on the association of substance use and facial injuries have been among men.[12] One study of subjects with mandible fractures found the ratio of men to women was 5:1; other reported ratios have ranged from 3:1 to 5.4:1.[13–17] Drinking alcohol not only is a risk factor for violent behavior but also may increase the risk of assault, especially for females.[18] In a study of female patients seen at a busy regional maxillofacial unit between 2000 and 2004, the most common mode of injury in alcohol-related incidents was interpersonal violence.[19]

Collectively, these studies implicate interpersonal violence as the "pathway" that links substance use and orofacial injuries. Research on substance use and violent crime has shown consistently that intoxicated individuals commit a high proportion of violent crime, including assault,[20–22] and that a majority of assault patients consume alcohol prior to assault, and sustain facial injuries ranging from minor cuts to severe fractures.[23–25] In a 5-year follow-up of 501 survivors of violent trauma seen at one hospital, Sims and colleagues[26] found that 62% abused alcohol or drugs. Using a case-control analysis, Vinson and colleagues[27] calculated the increased risk of intentional injury related to alcohol use and reported that drinking in the 6 hours prior to injury was positively associated with injury, with an odds ratio of 9.5 after 5 drinks.

The face is a common target for assault, and most injuries involve the mandible.[28] Haug and colleagues[29] found a 6:2:1 ratio among mandibular, zygomatic, and maxillary fractures. Specific to intentional injuries, Lee[30] reported that interpersonal violence accounted for 49% of mandible fractures treated over an 11-year period at one hospital's oral and maxillofacial surgery service, and that alcohol was a major contributing factor. Specifically, alcohol consumption was involved in 56% of all patients with mandible fractures and in 50% of all patients with maxillofacial fractures. In another study of maxillofacial trauma, of 246 patients treated for mandible fractures, the majority (53.5%) was caused by violent assault, and alcohol was a contributing factor at the time of injury in 20.6% of the fractures. In general, facial injuries associated with substance use frequently involve multiple fractures, and a high proportion of the patients end up requiring hospitalization and intensive surgical intervention.

## SUBSTANCE USE AND INJURY AMONG ADOLESCENTS

As with adults, the use of alcohol and drugs has been closely linked with injury in adolescents. Of all 13- to 19-year-olds admitted to a level I pediatric trauma center, 34% screened positive for alcohol or drugs on admission.[31] Another study of adolescents admitted for trauma found that 48% had positive blood alcohol levels.[32] Rivara and colleagues[33] found that 41% of 18- to 20-year-olds admitted for trauma had positive blood alcohol screens. The youth admitted for assault-related injuries were most likely to be positive for substance use, with a surprising 49% of the youth having behavioral evidence of chronic alcohol abuse. Similarly, Loiselle and colleagues[31] found that recent use of alcohol was more common among adolescents treated for intentional injury than those treated for unintentional injury. Finally, Murphy and colleagues[34] found that more than half (55%) of adolescents presenting at inner-city trauma centers with facial injuries had problem levels of substance use.

The strong linkage of substance use and injury found in the adult literature is also apparent in the trauma literature focusing on adolescents and young adults. In a comprehensive study of injury prevalence among adolescents in 35 countries, Pickett and colleagues[3] determined that poverty was positively associated with intentional injuries, and that alcohol use was positively and consistently associated with interpersonal violence, but not with school- and sports-related injuries. As noted earlier, in their study of adolescents presenting to inner-city trauma centers with facial injuries, Murphy and colleagues[34] found that more than half (55%) had problem levels of substance use. The orofacial injuries were predominantly intentional in nature, caused either through violent actions (ie, being in a physical fight with someone) or victimization (ie, being physically attacked). Moreover, a significant proportion of these youths (56%) had been previously arrested. Lee and Snape[35] reviewed trends in maxillofacial injuries over an 11-year period and found that males accounted for 88% of alcohol-related fractures, with 59% in the 15- to 29-year age group and 76% of alcohol-related fractures resulting from interpersonal violence.[35]

Recognizing that some of these markers can be used to identify at-risk adolescents and serve as the basis for secondary prevention efforts, organizations including the American Academy of Pediatrics now advocate that health professionals involved in trauma care be involved proactively in the identification of these youths. The fact that these adolescents are at high risk in several areas including substance abuse, reinjury, and arrest argues for multitargeted interventions as part of trauma care.

## SEQUELAE TO INJURY RELATED TO SUBSTANCE USE: COMPLICATIONS AND REINJURY

There are several complications related to substance use that can affect the healing process. Serena-Gomez and Passeri[28] found that patients consuming significant rates of alcohol per day had compromised recovery because: (1) this level of alcohol use suppresses T-cell counts and affects the body's responses in terms of cell migration, adhesion, and signal transduction; (2) the production of T cells is also affected, making the body more susceptible to bacterial colonization and subsequent infection; and (3) alcohol consumption negatively affected protein production, particularly collagen, and ultimately, wound healing. Of note, Passeri and colleagues[36] reported that patients using intravenous or nonintravenous drugs presented with postsurgical mandibular-fracture complications (ranging from 30% to 37.5% and 14.2% to 19%, respectively). Insufficient nutrition may also play a part in the recovery process of patients reporting alcohol abuse,[37] impacting both soft tissue and bone repair.

Substance use can also affect the outcomes of fracture treatment strategies, such as maxillomandibular fixation, that rely on the patient's ability to follow postoperative instructions and maintain adequate oral care. Shetty and colleagues[12] reported a significantly higher nonattendance rate among patients with facial injuries who had reported regular alcohol use at the time of hospital admission. Equally important, the behavioral precursors of alcohol and drug use that lead to violence and intentional injury also predispose vulnerable patients to recurrent injury. In the context of general trauma, hospitalized patients with alcoholism have been found to have a 16-fold greater prevalence of prior fractures than hospitalized control patients without alcoholism.[38] A 5-year follow-up of substance-abusing patients who were admitted to a level I trauma center in the Midwest evidenced an injury recurrence rate of 44%.[26] In the case of maxillofacial fractures, patients who return to a particular lifestyle are more likely to return with a similar injury in the future.[39] Of those trauma victims who survive their injuries, significant subsets (23%–52% of urban trauma patients) resume risk-taking behaviors, leading to recurrent injury or recidivism.[40,41] In their investigation of risk factors for reinjury in a sample of orofacial injury patients, Shetty and colleagues[12] determined that recidivist trauma patients, compared with sociodemographically matched cohorts, are more likely to report habitual

use of alcohol and drugs. Also, alcohol screening indicated that many of the patients were at-risk drinkers, problem drinkers, or alcohol-dependent drinkers.

All of these sequelae, both immediate and delayed, indicate the need for integrated care that extends beyond the management of the physical injury. However, implementing a collaborative care model is subject to several challenges.

## LACK OF PATIENT MOTIVATION FOR SUBSTANCE-USE TREATMENT

Most individuals who have an alcohol or drug use problem do not seek help or receive treatment. National surveys suggest that less than half of those individuals who had a psychiatric disorder (including substance-use disorder) in the past year received any treatment.[42,43] Estimated ratios of untreated to treated individuals have ranged from 3:1 to 13:1.[44,45] Simply put, only a fraction of individuals with substance-abuse–related difficulties seek or are offered professional help.[46] Reported reasons for affected patients not seeking treatment include not thinking the problem is serious enough, thinking they can handle it on their own, believing the problem may get better by itself, and not wanting to admit they need assistance.[47–49] Some patients think that the substance-abuse treatments may not be effective. Many of these reasons can be considered differential expressions of denial, which has been described as endemic to substance-use disorders.[50]

Specific to orofacial injury, Murphy and colleagues[51] found that 60% of patients treated for a facial injury screened for problem alcohol use and slightly more than 25% screened for problem drug use. Yet, only one-third of patients recognized they had a substance-use problem and of those, only 20% had actually sought treatment.

Even among those who do seek treatment, the substance-use patterns may be more established before they decide to seek help. Hingson and colleagues[48] determined that two-thirds of their respondents recognized that they had a drinking problem before age 30 years, but considerable time (1–2 years) elapsed between recognizing the problem and deciding to seek help. Most medically hospitalized patients with clinically recognized alcohol dependence are aware of their drinking problem, worry about the consequences of their drinking, and may even have thoughts that they need to change their behavior.[52] Patients hospitalized after a substance-related injury have been found to be motivated to change their drinking,[53] with aversiveness of the injury and perception of degree of substance involvement predictive of their level of motivation.[54] This ambivalence presents an opportunity for moving some patients toward behavior change.

## LACK OF TRAUMA CARE PROVIDER INVOLVEMENT IN SUBSTANCE-USE TREATMENT

Although a high proportion of patients treated for facial injuries has at-risk or problem substance use, screening by care providers is limited and very few receive referrals for interventions to cut back or stop substance use. It is not that care providers do not recognize a problem; in one trauma center there was an overall intoxication rate of 33% of 242 consecutive adult trauma admissions, and documentation revealed that staff had recognized it in 77% of cases, but only approximately 7% were referred to a treatment program.[55] There are several reasons why clinicians do not address substance-use issues. Multiple demands on their time is one common reason, a lack of training in screening and referral is another. In a random sample of members of the American Association for the Surgery of Trauma, only 54% of respondents screened 25% or fewer trauma patients for substance use, whereas only 29% screened most patients.[56] Those who did not screen were twice as likely to state that screening was not what they were trained to do and more often believed that screening offends patients. Therefore, a lack of training in screening, discussing, and referring patients for specialty treatment of substance-use problems is a significant barrier to comprehensive care of the injured patient with substance-use problems.

## SUBSTANCE-USE SCREENING IN THE TRAUMA SETTING

Screening is a preliminary assessment used to determine when an individual needs intervention or referral. There are reliable and valid brief screening measures to detect alcohol and drug use.[57,58] The World Health Organization (WHO) has developed screenings to identify a continuum of substance use and brief interventions,[59–61] and the Committee of the American College of Surgeons has supported routine alcohol screening and brief interventions in level I trauma centers.[62] This support derives from the strong research documentation; the growing field of screening, brief intervention, and referral to treatment (SBIRT) indicates that this method can reduce alcohol use.

There are 3 brief screens for alcohol or substance use that have strong reliability and validity. For adolescents (youths 14 years and older) the CRAFFT screen for substance use is recommended.[63] For adults, the WHO's Alcohol Substance Involvement Screening Test (ASSIST) is recommended,[64] as it has been found to be a valid screening for psychoactive substance use in individuals who use a variety of substances, and also who have varying degrees of substance use. In addition, the Alcohol Use Disorders Identification Test (AUDIT) has been found to be comparable, and often better, than other self-report screening measures for early-stage alcohol problems. In fact, for males an even briefer version exists (the AUDIT-C), which appears to be equal to the full screen.[65]

Recent research indicates that short, brief treatment of substance use in emergency departments can be efficacious.[66] The largest SBIRT service program of its kind was implemented by the Substance Abuse and Mental Health Administration in 2003. Of 459,999 patients screened, 22.7% were positive for a spectrum of use, and the majority was recommended for a brief intervention. Results strongly indicate that SBIRT is feasible to implement and there are significant improvements at 6 months for illicit drug use and heavy alcohol use.[67]

Most surgeons involved in trauma care agree that the trauma setting is an important venue for addressing harmful substance consumption,[68] and over two-thirds frequently check blood alcohol concentrations. However, the use of formal screening questionnaires is much less frequent (25%). Nonetheless, trauma surgeons are screening for at least alcohol disorders more frequently than they were 5 years ago. More effort is needed to get existing screening tests implemented through trauma centers for both alcohol and drug use.

## INTEGRATING THE SURGEON INTO COLLABORATIVE CARE

As stressed in the preceding articles in this issue, current trauma care is oriented toward tending to the visible manifestations of the injury, and only very rarely are the underlying risk factors considered. The traumatic experience of the facial injury may cause the patients to feel vulnerable and open to advice—the so-called teachable moment.[69,70] The injured patient may experience several concerns and fears, including permanent disfigurement, sustained recuperation with an effect on normal behaviors such as eating (eg, wired jaw), and shame. In such a vulnerable state, patients may be more likely to admit, discuss, and accept that they have a problem with substance use. This awareness renders them more receptive to reviewing their substance use relative to normative use, and to immediate feedback or referral to treatment for associated substance-use behaviors.

The patient's receptiveness to considering the consequences of his or her substance use, and the potential benefits of changing these behaviors presents the oral and maxillofacial surgeon with an opportunity to treat the patient more comprehensively. Longabaugh and colleagues[54] showed that the patient's injury and the perceived level of its association with substance use are predictive of readiness to change behavior. Warburton and Shepherd[70] have suggested that oral and maxillofacial surgeons are in a prime position to identify alcohol-related assault victims and ensure a coordinated multi-agency response to enhance the victims' chances of receiving comprehensive care and empathetic and informed assistance. Recognizing both the need and the opportunity, the American College of Surgeons has mandated alcohol screening among admitted trauma patients, for level I and II trauma centers. Because there is increasing evidence of the effectiveness of relatively brief substance-use interventions (some of which may be feasible even within the time, staffing, and financial constraints typical of busy trauma centers),[71–75] it is critical to change surgeon and surgical nurses' attitudes and behavior toward screening and brief intervention. However, several issues need to be answered so that substance-use screening, intervention, and referrals can become part of the care of patients with facial injuries. For example, how can oral and maxillofacial surgeons incorporate substance-use management practices into their workflow? Specific issues include: (1) setting about discussing treatment options with substance-using patients and determine which treatment options they prefer, (2) offering referral to substance-use treatment programs or other substance-use services to patients with active substance-use/abuse problems, (3) obtaining training in the skills required for screening for substance-use problems, and (4) integrating substance-use interview techniques into core surgical training.

## SUMMARY

Facial injuries are common, frequently result from substance-use–related behaviors, and typically involve the mandible.[76] Most facial trauma patients tend to be young, adult men in the 20- to 29-year age group. There is a strong need for service enhancement and service system collaboration and integration. The trauma care setting is an important entry portal into the substance-use care system, especially for uninsured patients who may have decreased access to other sources of medical care. Given the epidemiology of substance use among facial injury patients and the costs of providing care for recurrent injury and other attendant health consequences, the delivery of efficacious brief interventions and referrals for substance use by the oral and maxillofacial surgeon has the potential to have a large public health impact. Brief interventions have been shown to be successful in reducing substance use, and the best time for approaching patients about such treatment may be at the time of injury, when they are aware of the consequences of their substance-using behaviors. Most surgeons endorse psychosocial aftercare programs to reduce the risk of reinjury and promote patient compliance.[77] Thus, the care of facial injury patients calls for the use of brief screening instruments, and the integration of multidisciplinary expertise to address attendant substance-use problems.

## REFERENCES

1. National Center for Injury Prevention and Control. Injury fact book 2001–2002. Atlanta (GA): Centers for Disease Control and Prevention; 2001.
2. Danseco ER, Miller TR, Spicer RS. Incidence and costs of 1987–1994 childhood injuries: demographic breakdowns. Pediatrics 2000;105(2):E27.
3. Pickett W, Molcho M, Simpson K, et al. Cross national study of injury and social determinants in adolescents. Inj Prev 2005;11(4):213–8.
4. MacKay AP, Duran C. Adolescent health in the United States, 2007. Hyattsville (MD): Centers for Disease Control and Prevention; 2007.
5. Soderstrom CA, Dischinger PC, Smith GS, et al. Psychoactive substance dependence among trauma center patients. JAMA 1992;267(20):2756–9.
6. Madan AK, Yu K, Beech DJ. Alcohol and drug use in victims of life-threatening trauma. J Trauma 1999; 47(3):568–71.
7. Cornwell EE, Belzberg H, Velmahos G, et al. The prevalence and effect of alcohol and drug abuse on cohort-matched critically injured patients. Am Surg 1998;64(5):461–5.
8. Mathog RH, Toma V, Clayman L, et al. Nonunion of the mandible: an analysis of contributing factors. J Oral Maxillofac Surg 2000;58(7):746–53.
9. Ogundare BO, Bonnick A, Bayley N. Pattern of mandibular fractures in an urban major trauma center. J Oral Maxillofac Surg 2003;61(6):713–8.

10. Murphy DA, Shetty V, Resell J, et al. Substance use in vulnerable patients with orofacial injury: prevalence, correlates, and unmet service needs. J Trauma 2009;66(2):477–84.

11. Laverick S, Patel N, Jones DC. Maxillofacial trauma and the role of alcohol. Br J Oral Maxillofac Surg 2008;46(7):542–6.

12. Shetty V, Dent DM, Glynn S, et al. Psychosocial sequelae and correlates of orofacial injury. Dent Clin North Am 2003;47(1):141–57.

13. Bataineh AB. Etiology and incidence of maxillofacial fractures in the north of Jordan. Oral Surg Oral Med Oral Pathol Oral Radiol Endod 1998;86(1):31–5.

14. Ellis E, Moos KF, el-Attar A. Ten years of mandibular fractures: an analysis of 2,137 cases. Oral Surg Oral Med Oral Pathol 1985;59(2):120–9.

15. van Hoof RF, Merkx CA, Stekelenburg EC. The different patterns of fractures of the facial skeleton in four European countries. Int J Oral Surg 1977; 6(1):3–11.

16. Marker P, Nielsen A, Bastian HL. Fractures of the mandibular condyle. Part 1: patterns of distribution of types and causes of fractures in 348 patients. Br J Oral Maxillofac Surg 2000;38(5):417–21.

17. Sojat AJ, Meisami T, Sàndor GKB, et al. The epidemiology of mandibular fractures treated at the Toronto general hospital: a review of 246 cases. J Can Dent Assoc 2001;67(11):640–4.

18. Thornton DJA, Timmons MJ, Majumder S, et al. The impact of violent injuries on an NHS plastic surgery unit. Ann R Coll Surg Engl 2003;85(5):355–7.

19. Gerber B, Ahmad N, Parmar S. Trends in maxillofacial injuries in women, 2000-2004. Br J Oral Maxillofac Surg 2009;47(5):374–7.

20. Fothergill NJ, Hashemi K. A prospective study of assault victims attending a suburban A&E department. Arch Emerg Med 1990;7(3):172–7.

21. Koorey AJ, Marshall SW, Treasure ET, et al. Incidence of facial fractures resulting in hospitalisation in New Zealand from 1979 to 1988. Int J Oral Maxillofac Surg 1992;21(2):77–9.

22. Rix L, Stevenson AR, Punnia-Moorthy A. An analysis of 80 cases of mandibular fractures treated with miniplate osteosynthesis. Int J Oral Maxillofac Surg 1991;20(6):337–41.

23. Allan B, Daly C. Fractures of the mandible. A 35-year retrospective study. Int J Oral Maxillofac Surg 1990; 19(5):268–71.

24. Shepherd JP, Robinson L, Levers BG. Roots of urban violence. Injury 1990;21(3):139–41.

25. Wright J, Kariya A. Aetiology of assault with respect to alcohol, unemployment and social deprivation: a Scottish accident and emergency department case-control study. Injury 1997;28(5–6):369–72.

26. Sims DW, Bivins BA, Obeid FN, et al. Urban trauma: a chronic recurrent disease. J Trauma 1989;29(7): 940–7.

27. Vinson DC, Borges G, Cherpitel CJ. The risk of intentional injury with acute and chronic alcohol exposures: a case-control and case-crossover study. J Stud Alcohol 2003;64(3):350–7.

28. Serena-Gómez E, Passeri LA. Complications of mandible fractures related to substance abuse. J Oral Maxillofac Surg 2008;66(10):2028–34.

29. Haug RH, Prather J, Indresano AT. An epidemiologic survey of facial fractures and concomitant injuries. J Oral Maxillofac Surg 1990;48(9):926–32.

30. Lee KH. Epidemiology of mandibular fractures in a tertiary trauma centre. Emerg Med J 2008;25(9): 565–8.

31. Loiselle JM, Baker MD, Templeton JM, et al. Substance abuse in adolescent trauma. Ann Emerg Med 1993;22(10):1530–4.

32. Hicks BA, Morris JA, Bass SM, et al. Alcohol and the adolescent trauma population. J Pediatr Surg 1990; 25(9):944–9.

33. Rivara FP, Gurney JG, Ries RK, et al. A descriptive study of trauma, alcohol, and alcoholism in young adults. J Adolesc Health 1992;13(8):663–7.

34. Murphy DA, Shetty V, Der-Martirosian C, et al. Factors associated with orofacial injury and willingness to participate in interventions among adolescents treated in trauma centers. J Oral Maxillofac Surg 2009;67(12):2627–35.

35. Lee KH, Snape L. Role of alcohol in maxillofacial fractures. N Z Med J 2008;121(1271):15–23.

36. Passeri LA, Ellis E, Sinn DP. Relationship of substance abuse to complications with mandibular fractures. J Oral Maxillofac Surg 1993;51(1):22–5.

37. Sandler NA. Patients who abuse drugs. Oral Surg Oral Med Oral Pathol Oral Radiol Endod 2001; 91(1):12–4.

38. National Institute on Alcoholism and Alcohol Abuse. Screening for alcoholism in primary care settings. Rockville (MD): Alcohol, Drug Abuse, and Mental Health Administration; 1987.

39. Layton S, Dickenson AJ, Norris S. Maxillofacial fractures: a study of recurrent victims. Injury 1994;25(8): 523–5.

40. Redeker NS, Smeltzer SC, Kirkpatrick J, et al. Risk factors of adolescent and young adult trauma victims. Am J Crit Care 1995;4(5):370–8.

41. Smith RS, Fry WR, Morabito DJ, et al. Recidivism in an urban trauma center. Arch Surg 1992;127(6): 668–70.

42. Kessler RC, Nelson CB, McGonagle KA, et al. The epidemiology of co-occurring addictive and mental disorders: implications for prevention and service utilization. Am J Orthopsychiatry 1996; 66(1):17–31.

43. Wang PS, Lane M, Olfson M, et al. Twelve-month use of mental health services in the United States: results from the national comorbidity survey replication. Arch Gen Psychiatry 2005;62(6):629–40.

44. Cunningham JA, Sobell LC, Sobell MB, et al. Barriers to treatment: why alcohol and drug abusers delay or never seek treatment. Addict Behav 1993; 18(3):347–53.

45. Sobell LC, Sobell MB, Toneatto T. Recovery from alcohol problems without treatment. In: Heather N, Miller WR, Greeley J, editors. Self-control and the addictive behaviours. New York: MacMillan; 1992. p. 198–242.

46. Tucker JA, King MP. Resolving alcohol and drug problems: influences on addictive behavior change and help-seeking processes. In: Tucker JA, Donovan DM, Marlatt GA, editors. Changing addictive behavior: bridging clinical and public health strategies. New York: Guilford Press; 1999. p. 97–126.

47. Grant BF. Toward an alcohol treatment model: a comparison of treated and untreated respondents with DSM-IV alcohol use disorders in the general population. Alcohol Clin Exp Res 1996;20(2):372–8.

48. Hingson R, Mangione T, Meyers A, et al. Seeking help for drinking problems; a study in the Boston Metropolitan area. J Stud Alcohol 1982;43(3): 273–88.

49. Miller WR, Sovereign RG, Krege B. Motivational interviewing with problem drinkers: II. The drinker's check-up as a preventive intervention. Behav Psychother 1988;16(4):251–68.

50. Baekeland F, Lundwall L. Engaging the alcoholic in treatment and keeping him there. In: Kissin B, Begleiter H, editors, The biology of alcoholism, vol. 5. New York: Plenum Press; 1977. p. 161–95.

51. Murphy DA, Shetty V, Zigler C, et al. Willingness of facial injury patients to change causal substance using behaviors. Subst Abus, in press.

52. Stewart SH, Connors GJ. Perceived health status, alcohol-related problems, and readiness to change among medically hospitalized, alcohol-dependent patients. J Hosp Med 2007;2(6):372–7.

53. Apodaca TR, Schermer CR. Readiness to change alcohol use after trauma. J Trauma 2003;54(5): 990–4.

54. Longabaugh R, Minugh PA, Nirenberg TD, et al. Injury as a motivator to reduce drinking. Acad Emerg Med 1995;2(9):817–25.

55. Silver BA, Sporty LD. Behavioral correlates and staff recognition of alcohol use in a university hospital trauma service. Psychosomatics 1990;31(4):420–5.

56. Danielsson PE, Rivara FP, Gentilello LM, et al. Reasons why trauma surgeons fail to screen for alcohol problems. Arch Surg 1999;134(5):564–8.

57. Hungerford DW, Pollock DA, Todd KH. Acceptability of emergency department-based screening and brief intervention for alcohol problems. Acad Emerg Med 2000;7(12):1383–92.

58. Kelly TM, Donovan JE, Chung T, et al. Alcohol use disorders among emergency department-treated older adolescents: a new brief screen (RUFT-Cut) using the AUDIT, CAGE, CRAFFT, and RAPS-QF. Alcohol Clin Exp Res 2004;28(5):746–53.

59. Babor TF, Higgins-Biddle JC, Saunders JB, et al. The Alcohol Use Disorders Identification Test (AUDIT): guidelines for use in primary care. Geneva (Switzerland): World Health Organization; 2001.

60. Humeniuk R, Dennington V, Ali R. The effectiveness of a brief intervention for illicit drugs linked to the alcohol, smoking and substance involvement screening test (ASSIST) in primary health care settings: a technical report of phase III findings of the WHO ASSIST randomized controlled trial. Geneva (Switzerland): World Health Organization; 2008.

61. Knight JR, Sherritt L, Shrier LA, et al. Validity of the CRAFFT substance abuse screening test among adolescent clinic patients. Arch Pediatr Adolesc Med 2002;156(6):607–14.

62. American College of Surgeons, Committee on Trauma. Alcohol screening and brief intervention (SBI) for trauma patients. Washington, DC: U.S. Department of Health and Human Services; 2007.

63. Knight JR, Sherritt L, Harris SK, et al. Validity of brief alcohol screening tests among adolescents: a comparison of the AUDIT, POSIT, CAGE, and CRAFFT. Alcohol Clin Exp Res 2003;27:67–73.

64. Newcombe DAL, Humeniuk RE, Ali R. Validation of the World Health Organization Alcohol, Smoking and Substance Involvement Screening Test (ASSIST): report of results from the Australian site. Drug Alcohol Rev 2005;24:217–26.

65. Reinert DF, Allen JP. The Alcohol Use Disorders Identification Test (AUDIT): a review of recent research. Alcohol Clin Exp Res 2002;26:272–9.

66. Gentilello LM, Rivara FP, Donovan DM, et al. Alcohol interventions in a trauma center as a means of reducing the risk of injury recurrence. Ann Surg 1999;230(4):473–83.

67. Madras BK, Compton WM, Avula D, et al. Screening, brief interventions, referral to treatment (SBIRT) for illicit drug and alcohol use at multiple healthcare sites: comparison at intake and 6 months later. Drug Alcohol Depend 2009;99(1–3):280–95.

68. Schermer CR, Gentilello LM, Hoyt DB, et al. National survey of trauma surgeons' use of alcohol screening and brief intervention. J Trauma 2003;55(5):849–56.

69. Smith AJ, Shepherd JP, Hodgson RJ. Brief interventions for patients with alcohol-related trauma. Br J Oral Maxillofac Surg 1998;36(6):408–15.

70. Warburton AL, Shepherd JP. Alcohol-related violence and the role of oral and maxillofacial surgeons in multi-agency prevention. Int J Oral Maxillofac Surg 2002;31(6):657–63.

71. Bien TH, Miller WR, Tonigan JS. Brief interventions for alcohol problems: a review. Addiction 1993; 88(3):315–35.

72. Fleming MF, Barry KL, Manwell LB, et al. Brief physician advice for problem alcohol drinkers. A randomized controlled trial in community-based primary care practices. JAMA 1997;277(13):1039–45.

73. Fuller MG, Diamond DL, Jordan ML, et al. The role of a substance abuse consultation team in a trauma center. J Stud Alcohol 1995;56(3):267–71.

74. Greber RA, Allen KM, Soeken KL, et al. Outcome of trauma patients after brief intervention by a substance abuse consultation service. Am J Addict 1997;6(1):38–47.

75. Wilk AI, Jensen NM, Havighurst TC. Meta-analysis of randomized control trials addressing brief interventions in heavy alcohol drinkers. J Gen Intern Med 1997;12(5):274–83.

76. Laski R, Ziccardi VB, Broder HL, et al. Facial trauma: a recurrent disease? The potential role of disease prevention. J Oral Maxillofac Surg 2004;62(6):685–8.

77. Zazzali JL, Marshall GN, Shetty V, et al. Provider perceptions of patient psychosocial needs after orofacial injury. J Oral Maxillofac Surg 2007;65(8):1584–9.

# Orofacial Injuries as Markers for Intimate Partner Violence

Leslie R. Halpern, DDS, MD, PhD, MPH

## KEYWORDS

- Intimate partner violence (IPV)
- Maxillofacial injuries • Head
- Neck and facial injuries • Diagnostic protocol

Intimate partner violence (IPV) is physical or sexual violence made by 1 partner to another and is a prevalent and serious health risk, particularly for women.[1] It is estimated that more than 2.5 million women are abused annually and 30% to 50% of all female homicides were perpetrated by former or current intimate partners.[1,2] Beyond the physical and psychological repercussions, abuse victims have lower health-related quality of life and higher use of health services.[3] A growing awareness of the scope and effects of IPV have led various health care bodies including the American Medical Association and the American College of Obstetricians and Gynecologists to recommend that all female patients be asked routinely about abuse, regardless of their presenting injury or symptoms.[4] These recommendations are based on available evidence about the burden of IPV and the benefits of provider referral for help. Early recognition and diagnosis of IPV and appropriate referral may lead to early intervention to prevent future injuries.[2] However, there are no obvious clinical characteristics to aid in the diagnosis of IPV.

Current clinical standards for identifying IPV-related injury is patient self-report through either a spontaneous or a prompted disclosure. Other studies have suggested useful, but ambiguous, criteria for identifying victims of IPV seen in the emergency department and outpatient clinical setting.[5–7] When interviewed, only 1% to 6% of women report being assaulted by their intimate sexual partners. Whereas trauma to the head,

face, shoulders, breast, abdomen or extremities is often documented, the victim's report of injury is frequently incompatible or inconsistent with the mechanism or location of injury.[6,8–10] Facial injuries account for a significant proportion of emergency department visits, yet, few reports specify the causes or patterns of orofacial injuries in victims with IPV-related injuries.[7,9,11,12]

Interventions may prevent future IPV-related injuries, but they cannot be initiated until the diagnosis is made. The oral and maxillofacial surgeon is often the first and only health care provider to see these patients and is, therefore, in a pivotal position to help expedite acute care and referral for needed interventions.

This article presents data that support the use of orofacial injuries as a prime predictor variable in identifying victims of IPV and provides: (1) an overview of the epidemiology of IPV-related orofacial injuries; (2) a discussion of the role of head, neck, and facial injuries as markers of IPV, and their role as a diagnostic tool to facilitate the early diagnosis and referral for management of IPV; (3) a list of the advantages and limitations of using orofacial injuries as indicators of IPV; and (4) future directions to improve efforts to educate OMSs in identifying patients who are at high risk for an IPV-related injury.

## THE EPIDEMIOLOGY OF OROFACIAL INJURIES IN IPV

The prevalence of IPV-related orofacial injuries is underestimated. Although facial injuries account

Department of Oral and Maxillofacial Surgery, Massachusetts General Hospital, Harvard School of Dental Medicine, 55 Fruit Street, Warren Building, Suite 1201, Boston, MA 02114, USA
E-mail address: Lhalpern1@partners.org

Oral Maxillofacial Surg Clin N Am 22 (2010) 239–246
doi:10.1016/j.coms.2010.01.009

for a large number of emergency department visits, there seem to be few reports detailing the cause and pattern of facial injuries in women who frequent the emergency department/clinical setting. There has been a paucity of well-designed epidemiologic studies to measure more precisely the frequency of IPV-related orofacial injuries (Table 1). Motor vehicle collisions and interpersonal assaults have been recognized as 2 of the primary mechanisms by which orofacial injuries occur[7,13–25] although the etiology is dependent on the population studied. Injury sustained during interpersonal assaults is reported to account for 5% to 59% of all facial injuries.[24,26–28]

Interpersonal violence is a frequent cause of orofacial injuries[20,24,26,27] with most injuries occurring in individuals between the ages of 15 and 45 years.[11,22,25,29–32] An Australian study of 2581 patients with radiographic evidence of facial fractures found 1135 were secondary to interpersonal violence, 286 secondary to motor vehicle accident, and the remainder resulted from a variety of mechanisms. Most victims were male and the most frequently sustained injury was mandible fracture(s). Alcohol use was involved in 87% of these assault-related injuries.[29]

Reports from emergency department visits indicate that more than 75% of the time, women who presented with facial trauma had concomitant injuries within the oral cavity, especially in young adults.[18,33] Oral manifestations of sexually transmitted diseases (STDs), fearfulness of the dental examination, difficulty sitting or walking, and fear of the reclined position of the chair should alert the health care practitioner to signs and symptoms suggestive of physical or sexual abuse.[33] Through a prospective study of 203 adult patients seeking treatment of orofacial injuries at the King/Drew Medical Center in Los Angeles in 1998, Leathers and colleagues[34] found that a disproportionate number of women who presented with oral trauma (more than 38%) reported their injuries resulted from IPV. Similarly, a retrospective study of facial trauma in women by Huang and colleagues[9] in 1998 showed there was often inadequate documentation regarding the circumstances of the facial injury. The investigators concluded that IPV may be severely under reported in women presenting with orofacial injuries.

Case series reports indicate that 67% of women with facial injuries were assaulted by a husband or boyfriend with 68% of battered women in another study sustaining 45% of injuries to their midface.[10,11,13,25] A study by Ochs and colleagus[21] showed an extremely high incidence of head, neck, and facial injuries in victims of IPV. In their study, 94.4% of victims who identified IPV as the cause of their injuries had head, neck, and facial

**Table 1**
**Frequency estimates of maxillofacial injuries in victims of IPV[a]**

| Author | Design[b] | Dataset[c] | Age (Range) | n (%)[d] | Sex | Injury[e] |
|---|---|---|---|---|---|---|
| Zacharides et al (1990)[25] | Retrospective | Chart review | 18–92 | 51 (9) | F | H, N, F |
| Fisher et al (1990)[10] | Cross-sectional | Chart review | 10–78 | 23 (20) | F | H, N, F |
| Berrios and Grady (1991)[13] | Retrospective | Chart review | 16–66 | 149 (68) | F | H, N, F |
| Ochs et al (1996)[21] | Cross-sectional | Cohort | 18–51 | 15 (94) | F | H, N, F |
| Muelleman et al (1996)[19] | Cross-sectional | Cohort | 19–65 | 121 (51) | F | H, N, F |
| Hartzell et al (1996)[39] | Retrospective | Chart review | 15–83 | 7 (30) | F | Ocular |
| Huang et al (1998)[9] | Retrospective | Chart review | 15–45 | 100 (36) | F | H, N, F |
| Perciaccante et al (1999)[7] | Cross-sectional | Cohort | 24–56 | 34 (31) | F | H, N, F |
| Greene et al (1999)[17] | Retrospective | Chart review | 32 (mean) | 29 (22) | F | H, N, F |
| Le et al (2002)[11] | Retrospective | Chart review | 15–71 | 85 (30) | F | H, N, F |
| Crandall et al (2004)[30] | Cross-sectional | Chart review | 16–65 | 145 (72) | F | H, N, F |
| Halpern and Dodson (2006)[46] | Cross-sectional[f] | Cohort | 27–84 | 63 (31) | F | H, N, F |

[a] IPV, intimate partner violence.
[b] Study design.
[c] Dataset origin.
[d] n, frequency % injuries of IPV.
[e] Anatomic location of injury: H, head; N, neck; F, face.
[f] RCT, randomized controlled trial.

*Data from* Wilson S, Dodson TB, Halpern LR. Maxillofacial injuries in intimate partner violence. In: Mitchell C, Anglin D, editors. Intimate partner violence: a health-based perspective. New York: Oxford University Press; 2009. p. 201–16.

injuries. Nearly 35% of the women in this study who presented to the emergency department for treatment of orofacial injuries were victims of domestic violence. In this same study, if a woman had a head, neck, or facial injury she was 11.8 times more likely to be a victim of IPV than women who had other types of injuries. In the absence of head, neck, or facial injury, it was unlikely that the patient was a victim of IPV.

A study by Perciaccante and colleagues[7] evaluated head, neck, and facial injuries as markers of IPV in women. Of the 100 injured women, 58 had head, neck, and facial injuries and 31 of those were victims of IPV. A woman who had head, neck, and facial injuries was 7.5 times more likely to be a victim of IPV than a woman who had other injuries. Head, neck, and facial injuries were a sensitive but not specific indicator of IPV. The investigators concluded that women presenting to the emergency department for evaluation and management of orofacial injuries that were unrelated to motor vehicle accident should be considered at high risk for IPV.

In 1999, Greene and colleagues[17] drew conclusions similar to some of the studies previously mentioned. One-third of women with blunt assault facial trauma were subjects of IPV. Le and colleagues[12] performed a retrospective review of patients treated for domestic violence injuries. Eighty-one percent presented with orofacial injuries in which the middle third of the face was the most commonly injured area (69%). Facial fractures occurred in 30% and most of the facial injuries (40%) were nasal fractures.

Dutton and Strachen[35] examined the motives of men who committed IPV and interpersonal violence assaults against women seen in the emergency department. They concluded possible motives to be the need for power and the maintenance of gender roles in the assailant's relationships. The investigators suggested that assaults to the face and head reinforce the assailant's dominance and control by leaving visible wounds as reminders of their power.[35] The residual effect of injury, that is, scars, facial asymmetries, damage to dentition, loss of masticatory function, and psychological wounds, persist as painful reminders of the abuse.[36–39]

## OROFACIAL INJURIES AS MARKERS FOR IPV

Based on the accumulating evidence, our research group hypothesized that head, neck, and face injuries may be clinical markers of IPV.[7,13–25,40] Initial studies to develop an IPV diagnostic protocol using injury location, head, neck, and face versus other injury locations, were conducted more than a decade ago at Grady Memorial Hospital (GMH), Atlanta, GA. Grady Memorial is a level I trauma center serving a medically indigent population. Demographics consisted of 88% Afro-American, 7.6% white, 3.6% Hispanic, and 0.5% Asian. Ochs and colleagues[21] reported the initial findings based on a sample of 127 male and female subjects who presented to the emergency department for evaluation and management of nonverifiable injuries. The prevalence of IPV in this setting was 30%. Injury location was determined by physical examination and grouped into head-neck-face (HNF) or other. Subject self-reports were used to determine the cause of the injury. IPV victims were defined as those who reported that their injuries were a result of assaults by their intimate partners. The results of our initial study suggested that injuries localized to the HNF region were associated with an increased risk for injury as a result of IPV (relative risk [RR] = 11.8; 95% confidence interval [CI] = 1.65, 85.8, $P$ = .01). In this clinical setting, HNF injuries as markers of IPV had high sensitivity (94%), but poor specificity (45%).[21]

These results also suggested, consistent with other studies, that women were much more likely than men to be victims of IPV. The low specificity (45%) for ruling in an IPV-related cause prompted a second cross-sectional analysis of the same subject population that was limited to women. The purposes of this second investigation were (1) to confirm the findings of the first study and (2) to identify other risk factors for IPV that may improve specificity. The prevalence of IPV was 34%. HNF injuries were associated with an increased risk for injuries as a result of IPV (RR = 7.5, 95% CI = 2,5, 22.9, $P$<.001). Age was identified as a confounding variable as it was associated with injury location and with the cause of the injury. After controlling for age, injury location was still associated with IPV ($P$<.002). The results suggested that younger women with HNF trauma were more likely to be victims of IPV than older women with injuries to non-HNF locations (chest, abdomen, extremities). When injury location and age were included in the model, the combined sensitivity and specificity of these 2 predictors was 91% and 59%, respectively.[7]

In an effort to enhance the specificity of HNF injuries as objective markers for IPV, a third preliminary study was conducted in which 2 screening instruments were added: (1) short Woman Abuse Screening Tool (short-WAST) and (2) Partner Violence Screen (PVS).[41,42] A positive response to either the WAST or PVS was associated with IPV etiology. Combining injury location and the WAST or PVS score resulted in a diagnostic tool with

90% sensitivity and 93% specificity. The model was validated in an independent sample in which injury location and short-WAST score, when combined, were statistically associated with an increased risk of IPV than injury alone or use of the screening instruments alone (P<.05).[43,44]

Although the problems of IPV span cultural, socioeconomic, and geographic barriers, it was not clear that the proposed diagnostic tool comprising of 2 elements, injury location and response to the screening questionnaire, was applicable in different geographic or clinical settings. To assess the generalizability of the diagnostic protocol, the investigators implemented the protocol in a geographic setting with a subject population that contrasted markedly with the setting and sample used in the preliminary studies. Halpern and colleagues[45] tested the external validity of the protocol using the 2 variables of injury location and a verbal questionnaire associated with IPV-related injuries from the preliminary studies stated earlier.[46] By comparing 2 hospitals that differed by geographic location, socioeconomic status, and health care cost, their results suggested that clinicians can use injury location in conjunction with the PVS score to stratify (ie, as high or low) the risk of self-report of IPV-related injuries. Additional studies have determined that, in terms of detecting women with IPV-related injuries, the investigators proposed diagnostic protocol is 40 times more likely to report an IPV-related injury compared with 11 times more likely with the standard operating procedure of the emergency department (OR; P = .01). The sensitivity of the diagnostic protocol was superior to standard operating procedures, but specificities were equivalent.[47]

Other studies have identified age, race, income, education, and social history as risk factors for IPV-related injuries.[46,48] A recent study developed a predictive model using head, neck, and facial injury location and responses to a verbal questionnaire to stratify risk of self-report of IPV-related injury. This risk was modified by other variables of age and race and tested in a predictive model for goodness of fit using an independent set of patients to compare the model with. The investigators concluded that injury location, positive responses to the questionnaire, and age are associated with IPV providing a set of risk factors that may facilitate the early diagnosis of IPV.[46]

## LIMITATIONS OF SURVEYS USING OROFACIAL INJURIES AS RISK PREDICTORS OF IPV

Although the tool discussed earlier seems valid, there is still controversy on whether routine screenings for IPV should be performed in health care settings. The United States Preventive Services Task Force in 2004 found insufficient evidence to recommend for or against routine screening of women for IPV.[49] A systematic review was published in June 2006 to answer the question, "Should health professionals screen women for domestic violence?" Some of the papers in this review suggested that women respondents were often accepting of screening in the health care setting but health professionals were frequently not in favor of screening. A systematic review was published in the Cochran Database of Systematic Reviews in 2005 on domestic violence screening and intervention programs for adults who had dental or facial injuries. The investigators found no eligible randomized controlled trials on this topic. They concluded that "there is no evidence to support or refute the effectiveness of screening and intervention programs detecting and supporting victims of domestic violence with dental or facial injuries."[50] Yet, there are individual studies that suggest the value of screening for violence and abuse. Taliaferro[51] has written a review article on the topic of screening and identification of violence and abuse. She emphasized the need to assess risk versus benefit of such screening to individual patients. Although anecdotal evidence suggests the benefits of screening, there are potential risks to such questionnaires.[49,51]

Some of the limitations that often challenge assessment of screening tools are as follows.

### Selection Bias

Women who are recruited from the emergency department in a metropolitan hospital may represent 1 extreme population in the degree of abuse and socioeconomic characteristics than the population demographics of other hospital and clinical settings. The implementation of these diagnostic protocols in multiple clinical settings can control for selection bias.[44,52]

### Misclassification

Measuring the outcome variable (cause of injury) at 1 point in time and relying on subject self-reports may result in misclassification. There are 2 major types of misclassification: false-positives and false-negatives. A false-positive is defined as a subject who reported she was injured as a result of IPV, when in fact the cause of her injury was something other than IPV. False-positive errors occur rarely.[44,52] A false-negative is defined as a subject who reported an injury as a result of some other cause, when in fact it was caused by IPV. This error occurs more commonly.[53–67] The net effect of having predominately 1 type of misclassification error (false-negative $\gg$ false-positives) results in an underestimation of the true sensitivity and should have minimal effect on the specificity estimate.

## Limitations of the Diagnostic Protocol

The hallmark of a successful diagnostic protocol is to have excellent sensitivity, specificity, positive predictive value (PPV), and negative predictive value (NPV). It is therefore critical to set rigorous levels of these statistical criteria because of complications caused by false-positives or false-negatives (see earlier discussion). With respect to PPV and NPV, these are used most often to determine how successful a clinical outcome can be by identifying a disease with a diagnostic tool. It is thought that the higher the PPV, the better the clinical outcome. The studies that use injury location are characterized by high PPV and NPV compared with the standard operating procedures of the emergency departments that they were compared with.[40,44]

## Reproducibility and Generalizability

It is not clear that the results obtained in 1 clinical setting can be applicable to other clinical settings such as the private office or private community hospitals in the suburbs. The results obtained in 2 clinical settings that are markedly different in terms of their geographic and socioeconomic variables, as shown earlier, suggest that a diagnostic protocol using maxillofacial injuries and a questionnaire may be valuable in a variety of clinical settings. Other studies should include continued testing in different clinical settings to determine if the findings are repeatable. For instance, the protocol can be translated into different languages to allow early interventional strategies that will deter future battering of these and other future victims. Specifically, future studies should involve comparisons of ethnic differences in IPV prevalence rates to determine whether a culturally sensitive intervention can maximize identification rates of victims. Furthermore, because prevalence rates range from 5% to 35% in most emergency departments and 1 in 4 women who frequent the emergency department are victims of IPV, a closer analysis on differences in subject presentation with respect to chief complaint may also provide for a greater capture of victims of violence.

## EDUCATIONAL CURRICULA TO IDENTIFY RISK PREDICTORS FOR AN IPV-RELATED INJURY

In 2006, the American Dental Association news ran a commentary summarizing the importance of increasing the dental community's education, understanding, and obligation to recognize the signs and symptoms of family violence.[33,68] In 2008, the American Association of Oral and Maxillofacial Surgeons issued a consensus statement: "Oral and maxillofacial surgeons are dedicated to the health and well-being of all our patients, including those affected by violence and abuse, post-traumatic stress disorders, or traumatic brain injury." Education about violence and abuse in the training of OMSs and dentists, however, has been insufficient even when the signs of abuse are present. Zeitler[49] gathered data demonstrating that "dentists and dental hygienists are least likely… to suspect abuse in children, elders or young adults." Love and colleagues[69] found that "87% [of dental providers] never screened patients with head and facial injuries" and "18% did not screen even when there were visible signs of head and neck injury." Mouden and Bross[70] noted that "<1% of all child abuse reports are made by dental staff even though they are mandated to do so." Reasons for lack of identification may be divided into 2 types: (1) inadequate education on the approach to identify victims and (2) barriers to questioning that include patients accompanied by their partners and/or family members, cultural norms, and personal embarrassment by the doctor. Some dental professionals fear that there will be litigation if they are mistaken.[47,69,70]

Educational curricula for identifying victims have been introduced into the predoctoral and oral surgery residency training curricula of a significant number of dental and medical schools around the United States.[71] In 2008, Gibson-Howell and colleagues[71] published the results of 2 surveys: 1 sent in 1996 to associate deans of US and Canadian dental schools, the other sent in 2007 to US schools only. The surveys were forwarded to faculty members who taught a course on the topic of identifying patients who may be victims of violence and abuse. Results showed that 96% of dental schools included some curricula on child abuse; for IPV and elder abuse, however, that percentage was unknown. In dental hygiene schools, 70% had curricula on child abuse, 54.9% included elder abuse, and 46% included IPV. The topics relevant to the domestic violence part of the dental curricula included (1) the responsibility of health care professional, (2) the physical and behavioral indicators, and (3) prevalence. Critical questions were how these variables are factored into daily practice patterns, how IPV and domestic violence affect society (in terms of direct and indirect costs), and whether cultural norms influence the ethics of care.[71]

Several predoctoral education models are currently in place that can serve as case exemplars for intervention models. One model is based at Minnesota School of Dentistry. The Program Against Sexual Violence designed *Family Violence: An Intervention Model for Dental Professionals* for dental school and continuing education curricula. It educates dental professionals about the signs of abuse and neglect and teaches proactive and appropriate intervention. There are a series of DVDs available and continuing education is encouraged by the state.[72] As another example, at the University of California, San Francisco, Hsieh and colleagues[68] published results of a survey indicating that dentists have major barriers in screening for domestic violence, including having the partner at the office visit, a lack of training, and the dentist's own embarrassment. In response, the team developed the AVDR tutorial, an acronym for Ask, Validate, Document, Refer. The AVDR intervention was designed to help patients without imposing the unreasonable expectation that dentists solve the problem of family violence. "After taking the tutorial," the investigators noted, "dentists reported that they would be more likely to inquire about a patient's safety after recognizing injuries to the head or neck."[68]

## SUMMARY AND FUTURE DIRECTIONS

The oral and maxillofacial surgeon is in a unique position to expediently identify victims of violence and abuse and rapidly refer for further interventional care. In addition, the OMS should be instrumental in instructing other specialists (ie, emergency physicians, surgeons, general, and dental practitioners) to recognize the orofacial patterns of an IPV-related injury. Approaches include:

1. Applying IPV as a differential diagnosis of all female patients with orofacial injury.
2. A detailed injury history of orofacial assaults documented that includes mechanism of injury, weapon, relationship to assailant, description of injury, associated injuries, and history of prior assault.
3. Educating patients with head and facial injuries on the increased risk(s) associated with recurrent injuries; that is, co-occurring traumatic brain injury.
4. Encouraging referrals for IPV counseling including bedside danger assessment and safety planning before discharge.

Future directions for research could include:

1. Prospective clinical studies to further examine the sensitivity and specificity of orofacial and other injury types as clinical markers for IPV assault.
2. The use of clinical markers and patient profile data as indicators for a more extensive IPV evaluation; that is, other health disparities/chronic illnesses and how IPV affects the lifespan of the victim. Such IPV evaluation criteria could be a valuable adjunct to screening in some clinical settings.
3. Research to investigate the relationship between severity (contusion vs fracture) of orofacial assault injury and IPV lethality to expand the usefulness of facial injury as a clinical marker for IPV and better define the victim's potential risk.
4. Studies that examine the association between IPV assault orofacial injury and traumatic brain injury will aid health care providers and other professionals working with IPV victims and their family. IPV is especially prevalent in the treatment of military personnel returning from tour of duty with inability to readjust to their family/community.

## REFERENCES

1. Krug EG, Dahlberg LL, Mercy JA, et al. Violence by intimate partners. In: Krug E, Dahlberg LL, Mercy JA, et al, editors. World report on violence and health. Geneva (Switzerland): World Health Organization; 2002. p. 89–121.
2. Chiodo GT, Tilden VP, Limandri BJ, et al. Addressing family violence among dental subjects: assessment and intervention. J Am Dent Assoc 1994;125:69–75.
3. Melnick DM, Maio RF, Blow E, et al. Prevalence of domestic violence and associated factors among women on a trauma service. J Trauma 2002;53(1):33–7.
4. American College of Obstetricians and Gynecologists. Screening tools-domestic violence. Available at: www.acog.org/departments/dept_notice.cfm?recno=17&bulletin=585. Accessed March 31, 2010.
5. Knudson MM, Vassar MJ, Straus EM, et al. Surgeons and injury prevention: what you don't know can hurt you. J Am Coll Surg 2001;193(2):119–24.
6. Senn DR, McDowell JD, Alder ME. Dentistry's role in the recognition and reporting of domestic violence, abuse and neglect. Dent Clin North Am 2001; 45(2):343–63.
7. Perciaccante VJ, Ochs HA, Dodson TB. Head, neck and facial injuries as markers of domestic violence in women. J Oral Maxillofac Surg 1999; 57(7):760–2.

8. Spedding RL, McWilliams M, McNicholl BP, et al. Markers for domestic violence in women. J Accid Emerg Med 1999;16(6):400–2.

9. Huang V, Moore C, Bohrer P, et al. Maxillofacial injuries in women. Ann Plast Surg 1998;41:482–4.

10. Fisher EB, Kraus H, Lewis VL. Assaulted women: maxillofacial injuries in rape and domestic violence. Plast Reconstr Surg 1994;86(1):161–2.

11. Le BT, Dierks SJ, Veeck BA, et al. Maxillofacial injuries associated with domestic violence. J Oral Maxillofac Surg 2001;59:1279–83.

12. Monahan K, O'Leary KD. Head injury and battered women: an initial inquiry. Health Soc Work 1999; 24(4):269–78.

13. Berrios DC, Grady D. Domestic violence: risk factors and outcomes. West J Med 1991;155:133–5.

14. Cantril SV. Trauma system injuries - face. In: Marx JA, Hockberger RS, Walls RM, editors. Rosen's emergency medicine concepts and clinical practice. St Louis (MO): Mosby Publishing; 2002. p. 2766.

15. Centers for Disease Control and Prevention. Prevalence of intimate partner violence and injuries: Washington, 1998. MMWR Morb Mortal Wkly Rep 2000;49:589–92.

16. Flores C, Schwartz DT. Facial radiology. In: Schwartz DT, Reisdorff EJ, editors. Emergency radiology. New York: McGraw-Hill; 2000. p. 672.

17. Greene D, Maas CS, Carvalo G, et al. Epidemiology of facial injury in female blunt assault trauma cases. Arch Facial Plast Surg 1999;1(4):288–91.

18. McDowell JD. Forensic dentistry: recognizing the signs and symptoms of domestic violence: a guide for dentists. J Okla Dent Assoc 1997;88(2):21–8.

19. Muelleman RL, Lenaghan PA, Pakieser RA. Battered women: injury location and types. Ann Emerg Med 1996;28:486–92.

20. Nakhgevany KB, LiBassi M, Esposito B. Facial trauma in motor vehicle accidents: etiological factors. Am J Emerg Med 1994;12:160.

21. Ochs HA, Neuenschwande MC, Dodson TB. Are head, neck and facial injuries markers of domestic violence? J Am Dent Assoc 1996;127(6):757–61.

22. Petridou E, Browns A, Lichter E, et al. What distinguishes unintentional injuries from injuries due to intimate partner violence: a study in Greek ambulatory care settings. Inj Prev 2002;8:197–201.

23. Philip M, Sivarajasingan V, Shepherd J. Bilateral reflex fracture of the coronoid process of the mandible. A case report. Int J Oral Maxillofac Surg 1999;28(3):195–6.

24. Telfer MR, Jones GM, Shepherd JP. Trends in the aetiology of maxillofacial fractures in the United Kingdom (1977–1989). Br J Oral Maxillofac Surg 1991;29:250–5.

25. Zachariades N, Koumoura F, Konsolaki-Agouridaki E. Facial trauma in women resulting from violence by men. J Oral Maxillofac Surg 1990;48(12):1250–3.

26. Hussain K, Wijetunge DB, Grubnic S, et al. A comprehensive analysis of craniofacial trauma. J Trauma 1994;36:34.

27. Hutchison I, Magennis P, Shepherd J, et al. The BAOMS United Kingdom survey of facial injuries part 1: aetiology and the association with alcohol. Br J Oral Maxillofac Surg 1998;36:4–14.

28. Tanaka N, Tomitsuka K, Shionoya K, et al. Aetiology of maxillofacial fracture. Br J Oral Maxillofac Surg 1994;32:19–23.

29. Lee KH, Snape L, Steenberg LJ, et al. Comparison between interpersonal violence and motor vehicle accidents in the aetiology of maxillofacial fractures. ANZ J Surg 2007;77:695–8.

30. Crandall ML, Nathens AB, Rivava FP. Injury pattern among female trauma patients: recognizing intentional injury. J Trauma 2004;57:42–5.

31. Haug RH, Prather J, Indresano AT. An epidemiologic survey of facial fractures and concomitant injuries. J Oral Maxillofac Surg 1990;48:926.

32. Gilthorpe MS, Wilson RC, Moles DR, et al. Variation in admissions to hospitals for head injury and assault to the head. Part 1: age and gender. Br J Oral Maxillofac Surg 1999;37(4):294–300.

33. Kenny J. Domestic violence: a complex health care issue for dentistry today. Forensic Sci Int 2006; 159(Suppl 1):S121–5.

34. Leathers R, Shetty V, Black E, et al. Orofacial injury profiles and patterns of care in an inner-city hospital. Int J Oral Biol 1998;23(1):53–8.

35. Dutton DG, Strachan CE. Motivational needs for power and spouse-specific assertiveness in assaultive and non-assaultive men. Violence Vict 1987;2:145–56.

36. Sheridan DJ, Nash KR. Acute injury patterns in intimate partner violence. Trauma Violence Abuse 2007;8(3):281–9.

37. Craven D. Female victims of crime. Washington, DC: US Department of Justice; 1996. Report no. NCJ-162602.

38. Fanslow JL, Norton RN, Spinola CG. Indicators of assault-related injuries among women presenting to the emergency department. Ann Emerg Med 1998;32:341–8.

39. Hartzell KN, Botek AA, Goldberg KH. Orbital fractures in women due to sexual assault and domestic violence. Ophthalmology 1996;103(6):953–7.

40. Halpern LR, Perciaccante VJ, Hayes C, et al. A protocol to diagnose intimate partner violence in the emergency room setting. J Trauma 2006;60(5):1101–5.

41. Brown JB, Lent B, Brett P. Development of the Woman Abuse Screening Tool for use in family practice. Fam Med 1996;28:422–8.

42. Feldhaus KM, McLain J, Amsbury HL. Accuracy of three brief screening questions for detecting partner violence in the emergency department. JAMA 1997; 277(17):439–41.

43. Carey JW, Dodson TB. Predicting domestic violence based on injury location and screening questions. AAOMS [abstract]. J Oral Maxillofac Surg 1999;. 57(8)(Suppl 1):42–3.

44. Perciaccante VJ, Carey JW, Dodson TB. Injury location and Woman's Abuse Screening Tool scores as markers for intimate partner violence (IPV) [abstract]. J Dent Res 2002;81(Suppl):492.

45. Halpern LR, Susarla S, Dodson TB. Injury location and screening questionnaires as markers for intimate partner violence. J Oral Maxillofac Surg 2005;63(9):1255–61.

46. Halpern LR, Dodson TB. A predictive model for diagnosing victims of intimate partner violence. J Am Dent Assoc 2006;137:604–9.

47. Halpern LR, Parry B, Hayward G, et al. A comparison of 2 protocols to detect intimate partner violence. J Oral Maxillofac Surg 2009;67:1453–9.

48. Lipsky S, Caetano R, Field CA, et al. Violence-related injury and intimate partner violence in an urban emergency department. J Trauma 2004;57(2):352–9.

49. Zeitler D. The abused female oral and maxillofacial surgery patient: treatment approaches for identification and management. Oral Maxillofac Surg Clin North Am 2007;19:251–63.

50. Coulthard P, Yong S, Adamson L, et al. Domestic violence screening and intervention programmes for adults with dental or facial injury. Cochrane Database Syst Rev 2004;(2):CD004486.

51. Taliaferro E. Screening and identification of intimate partner violence. Clin Fam Pract 2003;5(1):89–100.

52. Brown JB, Schmidt G, Lent B, et al. Application of the Woman Abuse Screening Tool (WAST and WAST-short) in the family practice setting. J Fam Pract 2000;49:896–903.

53. Shepherd JP, Gaylord JJ, Leslie IJ, et al. Female victims of assault. J Craniomaxillofac Surg 1988; 16:233–7.

54. Shepherd JP, Shapland M, Pearce NX, et al. Pattern, severity and aetiology of injuries in victims of assault. J R Soc Med 1990;83:75–8.

55. Beck SR, Freitag SL, Singer N. Occular injuries in battered women. Ophthalmology 1996;103(7): 997–8.

56. Simo R, Jones NS. Extratemporal facial nerve paralysis after blunt trauma. J Trauma 1996;40(2):306–7.

57. Molitor L. A 26 year-old women with unexplained ptosis. J Emerg Nurs 1999;25(5):430.

58. Sorenson SB, Wiebs OJ. Weapon in the lives of battered women. Am J Public Health 2004;94(8): 1412–7.

59. Carrigan TD, Walker E, Barnes S. Domestic violence: the shaken adult syndrome. J Accid Emerg Med 2000;17:138–9.

60. Funk M, Schuppel J. Strangulation injuries. Wis Med J 2003;102(3):41–5.

61. Hawley D, McClane GE, Strack GB. A review of 300 attempted strangulation cases, part III: injuries in fatal cases. J Emerg Med 2001;21:317–29.

62. McClane GE, Strack GB, Hawley D. A review of 300 attempted strangulation cases, part II: clinical evaluation of the surviving victim. J Emerg Med 2001; 21:311–5.

63. Purvin V. Unilateral headache and ptosis in a 30 year-old woman. Surv Opthalmol 1997;42(2):163–8.

64. Covington DS, Wainsright DJ, Teichgraeber JF, et al. Changing patterns in the epidemiology and treatment of zygoma fractures: 10-year review. J Trauma 1994;37:243.

65. Ellis E, El-Atter A, Moos KF. An analysis of 2,067 cases of zygomatico-orbital fracture. J Oral Maxillofac Surg 1985;43:417–28.

66. Goldberg SH, McRill CM, Bruno CR, et al. Orbital fractures due to domestic violence: an epidemiologic study. Orbit 2000;19(3):143–54.

67. Abbott J, Johnson R, Koziol-Mclain J, et al. Domestic violence against women: incidence and prevalence in an emergency department population. JAMA 1995;273:1763–7.

68. Hsieh N, Herzig K, Gansky S, et al. Changing dentist's knowledge, attitudes and behavior regarding domestic violence through an interactive multimedia tutorial. J Am Dent Assoc 2006;137(5):596–603.

69. Love C, Gerbert B, Caspers N, et al. Dentist's attitudes and behaviors regarding domestic violence. J Am Dent Assoc 2001;132(1):85–93.

70. Mouden LD, Bross DC. Legal issues affecting dentistry's role in preventing child abuse and neglect. J Am Dent Assoc 1995;126(8):1173–80.

71. Gibson-Howell JC, Gladwin MA, Hicks MJ, et al. Instruction in dental curricula to identify and assist domestic violence victims. J Dent Educ 2008; 72(11):1277–89.

72. Short S, Tiedemann J, Rose T. Family violence: an intervention model for dental professionals. Northwest Dent 1997;76(5):32.

# Barriers to the Collaborative Care of Patients with Orofacial Injury

Eunice C. Wong, PhD*, Grant N. Marshall, PhD

**KEYWORDS**

- Posttraumatic stress • Collaborative care
- Barriers • Orofacial

Establishing collaborative care programs within oral and maxillofacial trauma settings may be an effective means of linking patients to the psychosocial services (ie, substance abuse, mental health treatment) that they need. Research suggests that orofacial trauma survivors may be motivated to address a range of trauma-related psychosocial problems during the period immediately after injury.[1,2] Moreover, preliminary evidence from general trauma settings indicates that collaborative care interventions show substantial promise in facilitating integrative care, which addresses the physical and mental health needs of patients with traumatic injury.[3]

A key step in designing and implementing collaborative care programs is to understand the potential barriers to the provision and receipt of mental health services within the targeted clinical setting.[4] Until recently, knowledge concerning barriers to psychosocial care, specifically with respect to patients with orofacial trauma, has been limited. This article highlights recent research findings from 3 interrelated studies on the patients' and health care providers' perspectives of the barriers in developing psychosocial services within oral and maxillofacial trauma care settings. In the first study, Wong and colleagues[5] examined orofacial trauma patients' receptivity and perceived barriers to psychosocial services for mental health problems. In the second, Zazzali and colleagues[6] explored provider perceptions of patient need for psychosocial services, and the barriers to establishing such programs within oral and maxillofacial

trauma settings. In the third article, Chandra and colleagues[7] examined the degree of concordance between providers' and patients' perceptions of barriers to psychosocial services. These studies were based on the interviews conducted with patients and providers at the Los Angeles County and University of Southern California (LAC+USC) Medical Center—a large level-1 trauma center catering to a mostly indigent population. Patients who were awaiting their 1-month follow-up visit at the oral and maxillofacial surgery (OMS) service for violence-related orofacial injuries were recruited. Providers included surgeons from OMS and otolaryngology. These studies answered important questions that are relevant for future efforts at establishing collaborative care programs in OMS settings. The following questions are addressed in this article: (1) To what extent are orofacial trauma patients interested in obtaining psychosocial aftercare services? (2) What are the key barriers to obtaining such services? (3) How cognizant are health care providers to patients' needs and barriers to psychosocial treatment? (4) What are some of the challenges that health care providers experience with respect to establishing collaborative care programs?

## PATIENT PERSPECTIVES
### Objective and Perceived Need

In general trauma care settings, only a fraction of patients with physical injury and documented mental health need obtain psychosocial

RAND Corporation, 1776 Main Street, PO Box 2138, Santa Monica, CA 90407-2138, USA
* Corresponding author.
*E-mail address:* ewong@rand.org

Oral Maxillofacial Surg Clin N Am 22 (2010) 247–250
doi:10.1016/j.coms.2010.01.001
1042-3699/10/$ – see front matter © 2010 Elsevier Inc. All rights reserved.

services.[3,8] Wong and colleagues[5] screened oro-facial trauma patients for posttraumatic stress disorder (PTSD), major depression, and alcohol use disorder (AUD) at the LAC+USC OMS service. A substantial proportion of patients showed objective mental health need with respect to meeting criteria for probable PTSD (34%), major depression (35%), or AUD (31%). Of those who met the criteria for at least 1 mental health disorder, 80% met criteria for at least 2 disorders and 50% met criteria for all 3 disorders. Despite significant levels of mental health need, only 8% reported that they were currently receiving mental health treatment. Moreover, of the patients who were currently receiving treatment, all had already been involved in mental health care prior to their injury.

Patients with a positive screen on any of the mental health disorders were invited to take part in an interview that inquired about their interest in receiving psychiatric aftercare and perceived barriers to mental health treatment. Patients were asked about whether they would be interested in an aftercare program designed to help patients who were injured in the face with anxiety, depression, and alcohol problems. Patients indicated whether they were very interested, moderately interested, or not at all interested in aftercare. Contrary to what might have been expected, patients expressed high levels of interest in receiving psychosocial aftercare; 48% expressed great interest and 36% expressed moderate interest in receiving psychiatric aftercare. Only a small proportion (16%) expressed no interest in psychosocial services.

### Perceived Barriers

Patients with orofacial injury expressing any interest in psychosocial aftercare were then asked about specific barriers that might impede their use of services. Patients were provided with a list of items representing different types of barriers (eg, financial concerns, lack of knowledge of available services, beliefs about the acceptability, and effectiveness of psychosocial treatment). Items were phrased as statements, and responses were provided on a 4-point scale ranging from 1 (strongly disagree) to 4 (strongly agree). Wong and colleagues[5] reported on the proportion of respondents who either agreed or strongly agreed that a given barrier might hinder their use of psychosocial services. On average, patients with orofacial injury endorsed a total of 7 different types of barriers. The 2 most highly endorsed barriers were lack of knowledge about where to find services (81%) and concerns about financial cost (71%). In addition, more than half of those who

were interested in psychosocial aftercare endorsed barriers related to transportation, insufficient information about counseling, wanting to handle problems on their own, and having competing responsibilities that would interfere with participating in treatment. About one-third of the patients with orofacial injury endorsed barriers that indicated ambivalence toward obtaining professional help for psychosocial problems (eg, not wanting to deal with problems, not needing any help). Barriers that were of less concern (ie, those that were endorsed by fewer than 20%) included fear of family disapproval, concerns about racial and ethnic discrimination, worry about what others would think, and child care responsibilities.

## PROVIDER PERSPECTIVES

Medical providers play a pivotal role in determining whether collaborative care interventions are successfully implemented and sustained. Coordinated efforts between medical, mental health, and support specialists are essential for the provision of integrated services for chronic medical and psychiatric problems. To better understand the views of medical providers for collaborative care, Zazzali and colleagues[6] conducted a Web-based survey with 20 oral and maxillofacial surgeons and 15 otolaryngology surgeons at LAC+USC medical center.

### Perceptions of Need

Providers were asked about their opinions regarding the need for psychosocial aftercare services, the adequacy of current psychosocial programs within their departments, and the potential for aftercare programs to reduce patient noncompliance and reinjury. Providers read a series of statements concerning these topics and rated how much they agreed with the statements using a 4-point scale (1, strongly disagree; 2, somewhat disagree; 3, somewhat agree; and 4, strongly agree).

With respect to the statement of whether there is a need for an aftercare program for patients that deals with their depression, anxiety, or drug and alcohol abuse problems, providers tended to somewhat strongly agree (mean, 3.46; SD, 0.70). Moreover, providers somewhat disagreed with the statement that hospital departments were adequately addressing the psychosocial problems of patients with orofacial injury (mean, 2.31; SD, 0.90). Providers also perceived benefits from psychosocial programs, including improved compliance with medical care (mean, 3.51; SD,

0.66) and reduced chances for orofacial reinjury (mean, 3.11; SD, 0.58).

In addition, providers were presented with various psychosocial issues including homelessness, depression, anxiety (eg, posttraumatic stress), drug abuse, alcohol abuse, major psychiatric illness (eg, schizophrenia), domestic violence, financial strain, unemployment, and legal issues. Providers were asked to rate the degree to which each psychosocial issue was seen as a problem in being a consequence of orofacial injuries, a contributor to reinjury, and a factor that interfered with patient compliance. Providers responded using a 4-point Likert scale (1, not a problem; 2, somewhat a problem; 3, moderate problem; and 4, significant problem).

Providers considered most of the psychosocial issues as problematic conditions that develop as a result of orofacial trauma injury. Anxiety, depression, and legal issues were rated as the top 3 problematic psychosocial issues that follow from orofacial trauma injury. Factors rated as most problematic in contributing to reinjury were alcohol abuse (mean, 3.77; SD, 0.43), drug abuse (mean, 3.74; SD, 0.51), and homelessness (mean, 3.58; SD, 0.72). Providers endorsed the same set of factors, that is, alcohol abuse (mean, 3.84; SD, 0.37), drug abuse (mean, 3.88; SD, 0.33), and homelessness (mean, 3.85; SD, 0.51) as the most problematic factors that interfered with patient compliance with medical treatment.

## Provider Perceptions of Barriers to Care

Providers were surveyed about various factors that may influence whether collaborative care programs can be successfully established in oral and maxillofacial trauma care settings. Specifically, providers were asked about how receptive colleagues and staff would be toward psychosocial aftercare programs, the ideal location for psychosocial aftercare services, and the barriers to implementing a psychosocial aftercare program within their department.[6]

With respect to the establishment of an aftercare program within their department, providers were asked about the degree of receptivity to psychosocial services from 3 different perspectives: themselves, other clinical staff, and administrative support staff. On a 4-point scale (1, very unreceptive to 4, very receptive), providers rated themselves as moderately receptive to the creation of aftercare services within their hospital department (mean, 2.51; SD, 0.98). In addition, clinical colleagues (mean, 2.14; SD, 0.77) and administrative staff (mean, 2.11; SD, 0.80)

expressed a similar level of openness toward aftercare programs in the department.

Providers were then asked to rate how suitable (1, unsuitable to 4, very suitable) the following locations were for situating an aftercare program: specialty mental health (social work and psychiatry), specialty surgical service (OMS, ear, nose, and throat, and plastic surgery), and community-based settings (religious institution, community agency, or free-standing independent location outside the hospital). Providers viewed specialty mental health (mean, 3.46; SD, 0.66) and community-based settings (mean, 3.29; SD, 0.52) as more suitable than surgical service settings for aftercare services (mean, 2.00; SD, 0.91; $P<.05$).

## CONCORDANCE OF PROVIDER AND PATIENT PERSPECTIVES

Collaborative care programs depend in part on providers' recognition of patients' barriers to psychosocial programs. Chandra and colleagues[7] examined the concordance between providers' and patients' perceptions of barriers to psychosocial aftercare within oral and maxillofacial trauma care settings. Providers and patients were given a list of 24 different items that reflected the reasons why patients might not attend a psychosocial aftercare program (eg, worried about the cost). Providers and patients rated the degree to which they agreed or disagreed with the statements (1, strongly disagree to 4, strongly agree). Patient-participants answered each item according to their own perspective, whereas providers responded from the perspective of the patients they treated for violence-related orofacial injuries. In addition, 2 items that assess factors facilitating the use of psychosocial aftercare were given. The items were phrased as statements relating to whether patients would attend an aftercare program on a doctor's or religious leader's recommendation.

Although providers and patients agreed on most barriers, there was significant discordance in the perceptions of the providers and the patients for about one-third of the barriers. In general, providers rated several structural and attitudinal factors more strongly as barriers to care than did patients. For instance, providers believed that lost job wages (3.1 vs 2.0) and childcare responsibilities (3.0 vs 1.9) would be even more of an obstacle to obtaining psychosocial services than did patients. For attitudinal barriers, providers provided significantly higher ratings than patients for the following items: problems are not a priority (2.9 vs 2.2), believing that counseling does not work (2.9 vs 2.1), embarrassment at discussing these problems (2.7 vs 2.0), believing these problems cannot be helped (2.6 vs 1.9), and not wanting to deal with these problems (3.0 vs 2.2).

With respect to factors that would facilitate the use of psychosocial aftercare, providers tended to underestimate their influence on patients' treatment-seeking behavior. Patients were significantly more likely than providers to believe that a doctor's recommendation would influence their participation in an aftercare program (3.1 vs 2.3, respectively; $P<.01$).

Overall, the findings suggest that providers are quite aware of patients' barriers to psychosocial aftercare services. In fact, providers viewed certain barriers as even more serious than patients. It seems that patients may be more receptive to psychosocial aftercare than may be commonly believed by providers. These results suggest that increasing providers' knowledge of possible misconceptions of patients' receptivity and barriers to psychosocial aftercare may engender greater motivation toward the implementation of collaborative care programs. Similarly, educating providers about the potential impact of their recommendations of psychosocial treatment to patients may be another fruitful avenue for increasing access to psychosocial services that are needed.

## SUMMARY

Oral and maxillofacial surgeons are in a prime position to target not only the physical needs of orofacial trauma patients but also the complex psychosocial problems that often co-occur. During the immediate period after an injury, patients seem to show an openness and receptivity to psychosocial aftercare services. Moreover, patients report that a provider's recommendation would significantly influence their use of psychosocial care. Collaborative care interventions may be well suited to capitalize on patients' and providers' interest in the required psychosocial aftercare programs. Although collaborative interventions are designed to meet the physical and mental needs of patients, they should also address major structural and attitudinal barriers to care. However, important provider barriers, such as the lack of financial resources and trained clinical staff, will need to be addressed before collaborative care programs can be successfully established. Further research is needed to determine the viability of this promising aftercare model in facilitating access to psychosocial treatment within oral and maxillofacial trauma care settings.

## ACKNOWLEDGMENTS

This work was supported by grant 5R21DE14973 from the National Institute of Dental Craniofacial Research and grant 5R34MH071569 from the National Institute of Mental Health. Authors also express appreciation to study participants without whom this study would not have been possible.

## REFERENCES

1. Gentilello LM, Donovan DM, Dunn CW, et al. Alcohol interventions in trauma centers. Current practice and future directions. JAMA 1995;274(13):1043–8.
2. Warburton AL, Shepherd JP. Alcohol-related violence and the role of oral and maxillofacial surgeons in multi-agency prevention. Int J Oral Maxillofac Surg 2002;31(6):657–63.
3. Zatzick DF, Roy-Byrne P, Russo JE, et al. Collaborative interventions for physically injured trauma survivors: a pilot randomized effectiveness trial. Gen Hosp Psychiatry 2001;23(3):114–23.
4. Katon WJ. The Institute of Medicine "Chasm" report: implications for depression collaborative care models. Gen Hosp Psychiatry 2003;25(4):222–9.
5. Wong EC, Marshall GN, Shetty V, et al. Survivors of violence-related facial injury: psychiatric needs and barriers to mental health care. Gen Hosp Psychiatry 2007;29(2):117–22.
6. Zazzali JL, Marshall GN, Shetty V, et al. Provider perceptions of patient psychosocial needs after orofacial injury. J Oral Maxillofac Surg 2007;65(8): 1584–9.
7. Chandra A, Marshall GN, Shetty V, et al. Barriers to seeking mental health care after treatment for orofacial injury at a large, urban medical center: concordance of patient and provider perspectives. J Trauma 2008;65(1):196–202.
8. Jaycox LH, Marshall GN, Schell T. Use of mental health services by men injured through community violence. Psychiatr Serv 2004;55(4):415–20.

# Social Support and Resource Needs as Mediators of Recovery After Facial Injury

Melanie W. Gironda, PhD, MSW[a,b,]*, Anna Lui, MSW[c]

**KEYWORDS**

- Social support • Social network • Measures
- Resource • Facial injury

Patients presenting with facial injury to trauma centers are invariably provided with immediate access to sophisticated surgical care. Yet, the antecedent risky behaviors and attendant psychosocial issues are not addressed by the trauma interventions. As discussed by Levine and colleagues,[1] patients with trauma are inherently predisposed to psychological and social problems even before the facial trauma. However, little attention is paid to psychosocial needs,[2,3] and any problems of posttrauma adaptation are largely ignored. Consequently, patients with facial injury receive little in the way of psychosocial support and interventions by health professionals during the recovery process. The care of these patients tends to focus exclusively on the repair of the obvious physical injury rather than the contextual issues that contribute to enduring functional impairments and diminished quality of life (QoL) and invariably to recovery. In recent years, medical professionals have begun advocating for the incorporation of psychosocial assessments and care in the management of patients with traumatic injuries.[4] One of the major contextual areas is that of social support and resource needs that influence recovery after facial injury.[5–7]

Ample evidence links social ties to health.[8–11] As a result, a US national committee of scholars identified *Personal Ties* as one of the top 10 priority areas for investigation that could lead to major improvements in health.[12] Social support is generally considered to derive from social networks. Berkman[13] defined social support as "the emotional and instrumental assistance that is obtained from people who compose the individual's social network." Others describe support networks as "the actualized potential of social networks that provide emotional and tangible aid."[14] Conversely, social isolation has been shown to contribute to poor recovery from illness and injury.[15] Unlike other physical injuries, facial injury may cause impaired communicative ability, sensory function, and alter facial appearance and self-image.[16,17] The face is the pathway through which an individual communicates and presents to others. Coming to terms with an altered facial appearance is a part of the recovery process.[18–20] Furthermore, diminished abilities to engage in social activities and social stigma as a result of facial injuries may result in a disintegration of social resources, which may further hinder the recovery process.

## EFFECT OF SOCIAL FACTORS ON REHABILITATION/RECOVERY OUTCOMES

In facial injury research, only a few studies examine the effect of social resources on recovery

[a] Division of Public Health & Community Dentistry, UCLA School of Dentistry, University of California, Box 951668, 10833 Le Conte Avenue, Los Angeles, CA 90095, USA
[b] Department of Social Welfare, University of California, Los Angeles, School of Public Affairs, 3250 School of Public Affairs Building, Box 951656, Los Angeles, CA 90095-1656, USA
[c] Department of Psychiatry, Veterans Affairs Greater Los Angeles Healthcare System, 11301 Wilshire Boulevard, Bldg 258, Room 115A, Los Angeles, CA 90073, USA
* Corresponding author. Division of Public Health & Community Dentistry, UCLA School of Dentistry, University of California, Box 951668, 10833 Le Conte Avenue, Los Angeles, CA 90095.
E-mail address: mgironda@ucla.edu

Oral Maxillofacial Surg Clin N Am 22 (2010) 251–259
doi:10.1016/j.coms.2010.01.006
1042-3699/10/$ – see front matter © 2010 Elsevier Inc. All rights reserved.

outcome. Often, the benefit of social support happens well after the patient is discharged from the hospital, when the patient begins coping with challenges of reintegrating back into work and social life. Patients with trauma often describe pervasive loss in multiple domains including physical, emotional, psychological, financial, social, and occupational functioning.[21] These losses greatly diminish the patients' sense of control and intensify their feelings of vulnerability. Correspondingly, researchers and practitioners are beginning to implement a perspective that turns the attention to people's inner strength and coping skills in being able to successfully overcome the psychological effect of adverse events and the ability to use available social resources to their fullest. For example, Wallis and colleagues[22] developed a treatment program for burn patients in a group setting to help them cope with emotional distress and to strengthen their social competence in dealing with disfigurement in public situations. The goals of these types of programs are to target specific factors and to either activate or strengthen resources that can affect prognosis or recovery, so that the patient is able to obtain social reintegration and improved QoL.

Perceived availability of social support and ability to seek help are important when confronted with a traumatic health event. Studies show that availability of social support and satisfaction with support is specifically associated with satisfaction with oral surgery and appearance postoperatively.[23,24] In addition, perceived availability of social support is also associated with fewer missed follow-up appointments for patients with orofacial injury,[25] a factor that is important in the case of treatments, such as maxillomandibular fixation, that depend on follow-up care.

In a study using qualitative focus group data of 50 African American and Latino patients with orofacial injury, Gironda and colleagues[26] examined social support relevant to the context in which vulnerable, underserved minority patient populations recover from their injuries. Availability of a confidant or someone to give good advice in a crisis provided respondents with the encouragement to continue with their recovery and meet the challenges that recovery posed, along with hope and a sense of purpose for the future and a sense that they were not alone. Male respondents found this support from their friends, whereas female respondents looked for a special type of confidant, one who they felt could relate to their experience and guide or counsel them through the recovery process. Male respondents, African American and Hispanic, were more inclined to discuss the positive benefits of having someone to give them

advice and emotional support, particularly the availability of a confidant. However, Hispanic women spoke about the lack of emotional support in terms of someone to understand and empathize with feelings of frustration during their recovery process. Another common theme was of sharing the burdens of care among family, kin, and friends. Help seeking in the form of instrumental support, such as help with meal preparation and transportation to clinic appointments, was provided by extended family. Although help seeking from formal, social, and mental health services were rarely mentioned, the use of the trauma clinic waiting area was identified as a venue for professional and personal support.

## PATHWAYS THAT MEDIATE BETWEEN SOCIAL SUPPORT AND PSYCHOLOGICAL ADJUSTMENT TO TRAUMA

Stressful and traumatic emotional stimuli, such as injury, accidents, or physical assault, can have powerful emotional effect independent of cognitive appraisal (personal interpretation of a situation). The concept of cognitive emotional processing, as first introduced by Rachman,[27] encompasses the mental tasks of contemplating, confronting, and integrating fearful or traumatic experiences into one's view of the self and the world for reaching emotional resolution. Failure to do so may result in prolonged cognitive (eg, intrusive thoughts, nightmares), behavioral (eg, avoidance, social withdrawal), emotional (eg, numbing, distress), and/or physiologic disturbances (eg, arousal, sleep disruption).[28] Social resources have received particular attention as a buffer against the ensuing psychological distress after traumatic injuries.[29,30] Fundamentally, the emotional adjustment to trauma may be facilitated by sharing the experience with supportive members, thus normalizing and desensitizing the event.[31] But, rather than the static view of social resources that serve as buffer against emotional distress, the social cognitive process model of adjustment suggests that how an individual reacts to their social network and available resources may help or hinder the emotional processing of a traumatic event.[32] **Fig. 1** illustrates an integrative framework of the interplay among negative events, life stressors, emotional adjustments, available social and material resources, and the psychological sequelae of trauma. Personal traits consist of hardiness and vulnerability (ie, self-efficacy, social adjustment, and limitations) that may influence or may be influenced by social and material resources, as well as life stressors (eg, financial hardship, conflicts), thus mediating the psychological sequelae of trauma.[33–35] Interpersonal

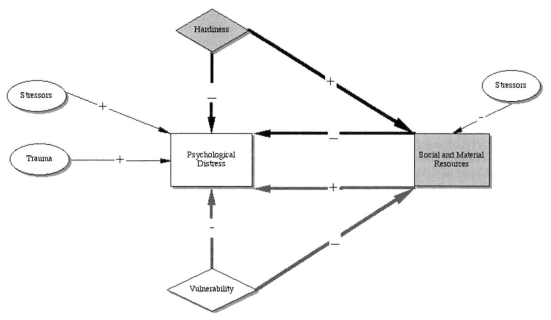

**Fig. 1.** Integrated model for stress, resources, and coping.

relationships are subject to individuals' appraisal and cultural norm. Social constraints may discourage individuals from thinking or talking about the experience, thus reducing opportunities for cognitive emotional processing and resulting in prolonged distress. For example, if the social norm is to avoid discussing negative events, even with members of their inner circle of friends and family, the opportunity for injured individuals to discuss their traumatic experience is diminished. Meanwhile, reticence of others to discuss the event may be interpreted as a lack of care or support, adding to the victim's negative self-image and self-blame. Furthermore, psychological vulnerability factors, such as avoidance and depression, may exhaust or deplete individuals' personal ties over time.[36–38] Fostering the existing strength within the individual and their social network through patient activation and motivational interviewing may moderate psychological vulnerabilities over time toward a more favorable recovery process.[39–41]

In clinical settings, the function of social relationships between people or groups and the resources obtained through these relationships is relevant to recovery. Trauma support groups can provide aid in developing effective coping strategies for managing the stresses they encounter during recovery and in strengthening familial relationships. Groups can also provide support for family members of patients with trauma and function as a means of developing social networks, thus serving to increase knowledge of and access to

community resources. Online support groups, chat rooms, or blogs have the potential to be the useful forms of social support and are beginning to be studied as a resource for support and information, particularly for isolated groups.[42,43] One example is the *Let's Face It* Web site, an "international support network for people with facial disfigurement, their families, friends, and professionals" based on a self-help philosophy (www.letsfaceit. force9.co.uk).

Neighborhood socioeconomics and the relationships between health care facilities and communities can have a serious effect on available material resources and help-seeking behaviors.[44,45] Received support generally emphasizes actual assistance and may sometimes be considered functional support, such as help with household chores, financial assistance, and the amount of time spend with others. Perceived support focuses on individuals' perceptions of the availability and quality of support they received. In a qualitative study of 29 patients with facial surgery, positive perception of emotional support from hospital staff was based on 4 components: staff approachability and concern, staff awareness of their needs, follow-up after discharge, and being given time to talk.[46] Unlike received support, which is concerned with direct supportive action, perceived support tries to capture individuals' appraisal of their ability to use support. Perceived support is believed to be strongly associated with self-esteem and self-efficacy. In the case of recovery from facial injury, an altered facial appearance may influence an individual's self-image, thus affecting one's perceived support.

Not only is the quantity of available support important, but the quality of the relationships has a critical influence on health effects. Levels of conflict, companionship, intimacy, and social skills inherent in any social interaction are important aspects of social support. Support is often viewed as a one-way street, with the assumption that social support is a constant resource independent of stress. However, some investigators[47–49] have conjectured that negative social interactions may have a stronger influence on the patients' well-being than positive ones and that life stressors and psychological problems can actually worsen the quality of social support and diminish its benefit. Researchers have identified 5 behaviors from family and friends that were meant to be supportive but are actually problematic to patients hospitalized for acute coronary syndrome: excessive telephone contact, high expression of emotions, unsolicited advice, information without means for implementation, and the act of taking over.[49] Similarly, not all social networks are conducive for positive health behavior, and some may actually foster negative health habits.[50] For example, in an evaluation of 12,067 cases followed between 1971 and 2003 as part of the Framingham Heart Study, researchers found that a person's chance of becoming obese increased by 57% if he or she had a friend who became obese, suggesting that this negative health attribute spreads through social networks.[51] The authors are finding that several psychosocial factors, such as low socioeconomic status, substance use, and mental health issues, are related to incidence and complicated recovery from facial injury[7,52]; so dysfunctional social networks and neighborhood/communities to which patients are returning may significantly influence the recovery process.

Aside from social resources, environmental factors, such as material resources and life stressors, also play significant roles in the social cognitive process. Life stressors, such as financial hardship, neighborhood disorganization, and unemployment, undoubtedly influence social and material resources. Nonetheless, careful evaluation of the hardiness of the individual and the fostering of strength in any given area of social and material resources may influence the recovery process in a positive way.

## IMPLICATION FOR CLINICAL CARE OF PATIENTS WITH OROFACIAL INJURY

The high resource needs of patients[5,7] with facial injury suggest a need for the identification of those at risk for poor postinjury emotional adaptation, both at the time of hospital admission and during follow-up care. Challenges related to time and resources in the evaluation of social support can be overcome with practical, standardized, and reliable screening tools, as well as careful planning and allocating of resources. Some practical concerns are (1) whether screening will be conducted through one-to-one interview or through written self-report, (2) the amount of time allowed for assessment given the clinical settings, and (3) the opportunities to repeatedly measure to capture progress during the course of the recovery process.

## MULTIDIMENSIONAL MEASURES OF SOCIAL SUPPORT

With ample time and resources, a standardized measurement that includes multiple domains of social support and social network would provide pertinent information about a patient's support system and resources (social capital). Good assessment tools should have a quantitative and a qualitative component. For example, knowing that a person is from a large family does not say much about how good the relationships are within the family. Although size is important, other aspects of the relationship such as frequency of contact and type of available support may be more important for a person recovering from a facial injury. Sarason's Social Support Questionnaire (SSQ), Cohen & Hoberman's Interpersonal Support Evaluation List (ISEL), Cutrona & Russell's The Social Provisions Scale (SPS), and Canty-Mitchell & Zimet's Multidimensional Scale of Perceived Social Support (MSPSS) are 4 standardized assessment tools that capture the multidimensionality of social support based on self-perception.

The Social Support Questionnaire[53,54] is a 27-item measure, but they also developed a brief version narrowing the items to 6. The brief version is comparable to the full version. Both test-retest reliability and internal reliability are psychometrically sound and has been used with normal population and subjects with serious mental illness.[55] Each item requires a 2-part response. First, respondents must list the people they can count on for support in given circumstances; second, respondents must indicate their overall level of satisfaction. This measure will yield 2 scores: the number of persons in their social support network and the satisfaction scores that range from 1 (very dissatisfied) to 6 (very satisfied). This measure provides (1) several perceived supports in a person's life and (2) the degree of satisfaction in several experiences with respect to well-being and self-esteem. The assessment is user friendly, and its brief version is designed for settings with time constraints and/or subjects with cognitive disability.

*Interpersonal Support Evaluation List*[56,57] is a 40-item measure rated on a 4-point scale that ranges from 1 "definitely false" to 4 "definitely true." This measure was tested and normalized with college students and generally population with excellent consistency and good test-retest reliability.[57] This measure was developed with the intent to assess 4 distinguishable support resources: (1) appraisal support, the perception of having someone to talk about important personal issues; (2) belonging support, the perception that he/she can identify and socialize with particular groups; (3) tangible support, the perceived availability of material aid; and (4) self-esteem support, the presence of others with whom the individual feels that he/she compares favorably. This multidimensional assessment has been used in several studies on social support and health recovery.[58–60]

*The Social Provisions Scale*[61] is a 24-item measure with a 12-item short form and a form that refers to specific relationships. This measure provides 6 relational provisions: guidance, reliable alliance, reassurance of worth, social integration, attachment, and opportunity to provide nurturance. These provisions are based on Weiss's[62] typology of loneliness. Emotional loneliness results from the lack of intimate attachment to another person and social loneliness from the lack of social network for the purpose of sharing interests and activities with friends and acquaintances. Like many social support instruments, it was designed to evaluate social support in the context of mental health outcome. However, during the years, this measure has also been used in medical research on coping with cancer and other chronic illnesses.[63–66]

*The Multidimensional Scale of Perceived Social Support*[67] is a 12-item scale that measures perceived support from friends, family, and a significant other. The reliability, validity, and factor structure have been demonstrated across different samples with excellent psychometrics.[68] The advantage of this tool is its brevity and simplicity, because it was designed with adolescents in mind, and it has also been normalized with psychiatric outpatients. Respondents answer items on a 7-point Likert-type scale (from very strongly disagree to very strongly agree). The limitation of this measure is its lack of domains on interpersonal resources and self-appraisal; however, depending on the inquiry, the MSPSS is direct and therefore easy to interpret.

The 4 instruments discussed earlier are related to the individuals' assessment of their relationships with others on the domains of satisfaction, intimacy, conflict, and security. Perceived support has a direct positive relationship to mental status, and therefore, it captures not only the characteristics of the relationships but also, to some extend, their personality traits. For example, in the SSQ, the reported number of supportive people may not have a direct relationship to the perception of satisfaction. Respondents may have no one they could name to count on for certain aspect but may be completely satisfied with no support in that area. Perceived support is shaped by the underlying personal traits or symptoms that are related to psychological distress. Therefore, one must interpret the data collected from these multidimensional self-assessments with careful consideration. Because it encompasses multiple domains, computing a weighted average across all domains magnifies the personality variance and frankly defeats the purpose of using a multidimensional tool.

The most commonly used measure for behavior-based supports is the *Inventory of Socially Supportive Behaviors* (ISSB).[69] The ISSB is a 40-item measure that uses frequency to assess the amount of support received in 4 essential functional areas. Function 1 is direct guidance, which includes offering advice, information, or instruction and also providing feedback about their behaviors, thoughts, or feelings; function 2 is nondirect social exchange, which is similar to traditional nondirective counseling behaviors such as listening, and expression esteem, caring, and understanding; function 3 is positive social exchange, which includes engaging in social interactions for fun and relaxation; and function 4 is tangible assistance, which includes material aids such as money or physical objects or sharing of tasks through physical labor. The ISSB has sound internal consistency and good test-retest reliability.[69] The weakness in the construct for received support is the lack of empirical evidence on its relationships to health outcome. However, it could also be that psychosocial intervention researchers favor perceived support because of its proximity to mental health; therefore less empirical evidence is established on the effect of received support on the health recovery process.

One commonly used instrument to assess social integration and screen for social isolation is the *Lubben Social Network Scale*, designed to measure perceived social support received by family and friends, which typically takes 5 to 10 minutes to complete.[70] Scores on the LSNS are obtained from an equally weighted sum of

10 items, each of which range in value from 0 to 5, resulting in a total score ranging from 0 to 50. A score of 30 or higher indicates good social network function. An updated version of the LSNS (LSNS-6) is composed of a total of 6 items designed to gauge perceived emotional and tangible support and actual network size by measuring perceived social support received by family and nonkin networks.[71] Scores on the LSNS-6 are obtained from an equally weighted sum of 6 items, each of which range in value from 0 to 5, resulting in a total score ranging from 0 to 30. Because of its brevity, it could easily be used in a variety of health care settings.[72,73]

## PERSONAL AND MATERIAL RESOURCE MEASURES

Aside from social resources, material resources may also provide the clinician a mechanism to evaluate the strength that may assist the recovery process. Material resources are often captured using QoL measures. Clinicians may glean from selected questions or subscales from these measures to determine possible areas of strength and deficits, useful for monitoring treatment progress. For example, Katschnig and colleagues' *Quality of Life in Mental Disorders 2nd Edition*[74,75] covers the entire spectrum of QoL issues, including QoL in specific mental health disorders, and treatment and clinical management issues. To assess individuals' perception of their social and material resources and adjustment to limitations in these areas, Weissman and Bothwell's[76] *Self-report Social Adjustment Scale* provides a brief measure, ideal when time is limited.

## SUMMARY

Recovery from orofacial injury is often a long process, requiring support from a broad network of personal- and community-based systems. This article presents a sample of assessment tools appropriate for clinical settings to determine social support and resource needs and to examine the role social support plays in recovery after facial injury. Determining social support needs should happen as close to the beginning of treatment as possible, allowing time to put in place the best possible social support network than wait until a patient is 1 step out the door to a less than adequate social network system.

Although minority populations disproportionately suffer from facial injury and are disproportionately high users of primary care services, their use of social and mental health services is low,[77,78] especially among patients with facial injury.[7] Oral health

care providers can play a pivotal role in strengthening personal and social ties that facilitate recovery by examining what aspects of social support help people to reach their full potential in spite of personal and environmental stressors. Patients with extensive facial surgery must return for follow-up visits to check wound healing or to make sure bones are healing correctly. This is an optimal time for social workers and other health care professionals to screen for social isolation and identify untapped sources of support and social capital from social networks of family, friends, neighbors, and the larger community.

To reduce the deleterious psychological and health effect due to traumatic injuries, health care professional may consider the inclusion of psychosocial supportive intervention, which may include screening, evaluation, and aiding the patient and family members in identifying available community and material resources they might qualify for immediately or in the future. In addition, anticipatory guidance may be useful, focusing on the potential loss of resources that patients with trauma can expect during recovery. QoL assessments related to job stability, financial resource stores, and available family and social support can help patients with trauma and their family members comprehend the difficulties they may encounter during the recovery period. Clinicians should be aware of cultural differences and if possible consider whether these differences may interfere with resources. For example, some cultural groups may assign stigma against persons with facial injuries, and therefore increase the risk of rebuke and self-blame. Less apparent are cultural norms regarding the use of public assistance and the process of applying for a disability bus pass or disability benefits as embarrassing or humiliating. Their refusal for public assistance may be viewed as a strength within their cultural group, but without careful evaluation, the lack of such resources may interfere with their QoL and their continuation of medical care.

### Resilience/Hardiness

No discussion of social support and resources for recovery from traumatic injury is complete without noting that not all injured persons suffer from psychosocial distress.[79–81] It is not that many do not suffer from the disturbing reactions of acute traumatic events, rather it is that the distress does not persist or manifest as posttraumatic stress. In a study examining hardiness and social support among African American and Hispanic subjects recovering from jaw fractures, 3 aspects of resiliency—(1) control, a sense of being capable of changing events; (2) commitment, a sense of purpose and active involvement in various work, social, and family activities; and (3) challenge, the perspective that change is normal and can be an opportunity for growth—were explored.[27] The recovery process of an orofacial injury presents ample opportunity for clinicians to play a pivotal role in strengthening personal and social structures that promote resilience or hardiness. To begin with, it is essential to examine what aspects of hardiness and social support help people to reach their full potential in spite of personal and environmental stressors. Patients with either jaw wiring or surgical plates must return for follow-up visits primarily to check wound healing and to make sure the jawbones heal correctly. This is an optimal time for health care professionals to identify social and material resources that foster hardiness. During follow-up visits, healthcare professional could ask patients whether there is anything they have learned or can learn from this experience. This is a way to identify areas that were perceived as a challenge and an opportunity to label and acknowledge personal growth that may have ensued. Another way to foster hardiness is to provide an opportunity for the patient to commit to follow through on a specific task in the process of recovery. The discharge plan is an ideal tool for partnership between the patient and the health provider to problem-solve difficult parts of recovery. One strategy is for the patient to identify a plan for the event in which wires become bothersome or pain becomes too much to take before it actually happens. Adopting health-promoting behaviors such as this empower the patient as an active and invested participant in the postoperative, recovery phase. Offering praise and reinforcement to the patient for figuring out effective, proactive, and creative solutions to the problems encountered will enhance patient's self-efficacy. Such encouragement not only sends the message that the patient's input matters and is heard by health professionals but also contributes to the patient's sense of control. Patient may further develop self-monitoring tools and coping skills if they are encouraged by their health professionals to review challenging and positive aspects of the recovery, such as those that went smoother than expected. The investment in fostering health-promoting behaviors and a strength-based focus in recovery can have a lasting effect for the individual to long past the recovery process.

## REFERENCES

1. Levine E, Degutis L, Pruzinsky T, et al. Quality of life and facial trauma: psychological and body image effects. Ann Plast Surg 2005;54(5):502–10.

2. Van Loey NE, Faber AW, Taal LA. A European hospital survey to determine the extent of psychological services offered to patients with severe burns. Burns 2001;27(1):23–31.

3. Thompson A, Kent G. Adjusting to disfigurement: processes involved in dealing with being visibly different. Clin Psychol Rev 2001;21(5):663–82.

4. Zatzick DF, Roy-Byrne PP. From bedside to bench: how the epidemiology of clinical practice can inform the secondary prevention of PTSD. Psychiatr Serv 2006;57(12):1726–30.

5. Asarnow JR, Glynn SM, Asarnow R, et al. Mental health needs of inner-city, orofacial injury patients. Int J Oral Biol 1999;24:31–5.

6. Glynn SM, Asarnow JR, Asarnow R, et al. Orofacial injury and development of acute PTSD. Int J Oral Biol 1999;24:26–30.

7. Lento J, Glynn S, Shetty V, et al. Psychologic functioning and needs of indigent patients with facial injury: a prospective controlled study. J Oral Maxillofac Surg 2004;62(8):925–32.

8. Avlund K, Lund R, Holstein BE, et al. The impact of structural and functional characteristics of social relations as determinants of functional decline. J Gerontol B Psychol Sci Soc Sci 2004;59B(1):S44–51.

9. Berkman LF, Glass T, Brissette I, et al. From social integration to health: Durkheim in the new millennium. Special Issue: XVth International Conference on the Social Sciences & Medicine: Societies and Health in Transition. Soc Sci Med 2000;51(6):843–57.

10. Bosworth HB, Schaie KW. The relationship of social environment, social networks, and health outcomes in the Seattle longitudinal study: two analytical approaches. J Gerontol B Psychol Sci Soc Sci 1997;52B(5):P197–205.

11. Lin N, Ye X, Ensel WM. Social support and depressed mood: a structural analysis. J Health Soc Behav 1999;40(4):344–59.

12. National Research Council. New horizons in health: an integrative approach. Washington, DC: National Academy Press; 2001.

13. Berkman LF. Assessing the physical health effects of social networks and social support. Annu Rev Public Health 1984;5:413–32.

14. Phillipson C. Transitions from work to retirement: changing experiences of older workers in the twenty-first century. Tijdschr Gerontol Geriatr 2004;35(4):146.

15. Peat G, Thomas E, Handy J, et al. Social networks and pain interference with daily activities in middle and old age. Pain 2004;112(3):397–405.

16. Cunningham SJ. The psychology of facial appearance. Dent Update 1999;26(10):438–43.

17. Rankin M, Borah G. National plastic surgical nursing survey. Plast Surg Nurs 2006;26(4):178–83.

18. Dropkin MJ. Coping with disfigurement/dysfunction and length of hospital stay after head and neck cancer surgery. ORL Head Neck Nurs 1997;15(1):22–6.

19. Lansdown R. Visibly different: coping with disfigurement. Oxford (UK): Oxford University Press: Hodder Arnold; 1997.

20. Robinson E, Rumsey N, Partridge J. An evaluation of the impact of social interaction skills training for facially disfigured people. Br J Plast Surg 1996; 49(5):281–9.

21. Cox J, Davies DR, Burlingame GM, et al. Effectiveness of a trauma/grief-focused group intervention: a qualitative study with war-exposed Bosnian adolescents. Int J Group Psychother 2007;57(3):319–45.

22. Wallis H, Renneberg B, Ripper S, et al. Emotional distress and psychosocial resources in patients recovering from severe burn injury. J Burn Care Res 2006;27(5):734–41.

23. Holman AR, Brumer S, Ware WH, et al. The impact of interpersonal support on patient satisfaction with orthognathic surgery. J Oral Maxillofac Surg 1995; 53(11):1289–97 [discussion: 1297–89].

24. Chen B, Zhang ZK, Wang X. Factors influencing postoperative satisfaction of orthognathic surgery patients. Int J Adult Orthodon Orthognath Surg 2002;17(3):217–22.

25. Brown KA, Shetty V, Delrahim S, et al. Correlates of missed appointments in orofacial injury patients. Oral Surg Oral Med Oral Pathol Oral Radiol Endod 1999;87(4):405–10.

26. Gironda MW, Der-Martirosian C, Abrego M, et al. A qualitative study of hardiness and social support among underserved, inner-city minority adults recovering from oral surgery. Soc Work Health Care 2006;43(4):29–51.

27. Rachman S. Emotional processing. Behav Res Ther 1980;18(1):51–60.

28. Foa EB, Riggs DS, Gershuny BS. Arousal, numbing, and intrusion: symptom structure of PTSD following assault. Am J Psychiatry 1995;152(1):116–20.

29. Hobfoll SE. Traumatic stress: a theory based on rapid loss of resources. Anxiety Research 1991; 4(3):187–97.

30. Hobfoll SE, Vaux A. Social support: social resources and social context. New York: Free Press; 1993.

31. Foa EB, Kozak MJ. Emotional processing of fear: exposure to corrective information. Psychol Bull 1986;99(1):20–35.

32. Lepore SJ. A social-cognitive processing model of emotional adjustment to cancer. Washington, DC: American Psychological Association; 2001.

33. Chun C-A, Moos RH, Cronkite RC. Culture: a fundamental context for the stress and coping paradigm. Dallas (TX): Spring Publications; 2006.

34. Holahan CJ, Moos RH. Life stress and health: personality, coping, and family support in stress resistance. J Pers Soc Psychol 1985;49(3):739–47.

35. Holahan CJ, Moos RH. Personality, coping, and family resources in stress resistance: a longitudinal analysis. J Pers Soc Psychol 1986;51(2):389–95.

36. Kaniasty K, Norris FH. A test of the social support deterioration model in the context of natural disaster. J Pers Soc Psychol 1993;64(3):395–408.

37. Lepore SJ, Evans GW, Schneider ML. Dynamic role of social support in the link between chronic stress and psychological distress. J Pers Soc Psychol 1991;61(6):899–909.

38. Lin N, Ensel WM. Depression-mobility and its social etiology: the role of life events and social support. J Health Soc Behav 1984;25(2):176–88.

39. Thew M, McKenna J. Lifestyle management in health and social care. Malden (MA): Blackwell Publishing; 2008. p. 261.

40. Cox WM, Klinger E. Handbook of motivational counseling: concepts, approaches, and assessment. New York: John Wiley & Sons Ltd; 2004. p. 515.

41. Miller WR, Rollnick S. Motivational interviewing: preparing people for change. 2nd edition. New York: Guilford Press; 2002. p. 428.

42. Davison KP, Pennebaker JW, Dickerson SS. Who talks? The social psychology of illness support groups. Am Psychol 2000;55(2):205–17.

43. Jerome LW, DeLeon PH, James LC, et al. The coming of age of telecommunications in psychological research and practice. Am Psychol 2000;55(4): 407–21.

44. Derose KP, Varda DM. Social capital and health care access: a systematic review. Med Care Res Rev 2009;66(3):272–306.

45. Kawachi I, Subramanian SV. Neighbourhood influences on health. J Epidemiol Community Health 2007;61(1):3–4.

46. Furness PJ. Exploring supportive care needs and experiences of facial surgery patients. Br J Nurs 2005;14(12):641–5.

47. Rook KS. The negative side of social interaction: impact on psychological well-being. J Pers Soc Psychol 1984;46(5):1097–108.

48. Rook KS. Social support versus companionship: effects on life stress, loneliness, and evaluations by others. J Pers Soc Psychol 1987;52(6):1132–47.

49. Boutin-Foster C. In spite of good intentions: patients' perspectives on problematic social support interactions. Health Qual Life Outcomes 2005;3:52.

50. Carpiano RM. Actual or potential neighborhood resources and access to them: testing hypotheses of social capital for the health of female caregivers. Soc Sci Med 2008;67(4):568–82.

51. Christakis NA, Fowler JH. The spread of obesity in a large social network over 32 years. N Engl J Med 2007;357(4):370–9.

52. Pattussi MP, Hardy R, Sheiham A. Neighborhood social capital and dental injuries in Brazilian adolescents. Am J Public Health 2006;96(8):1462–8.

53. Sarason IG, Levine HM, Basham RB, et al. Assessing social support: the Social Support Questionnaire. J Pers Soc Psychol 1983;44(1):127–39.

54. Sarason IG, Sarason BR, Shearin EN, et al. A brief measure of social support: practical and theoretical implications. J Soc Pers Relat 1987;4(4):497–510.

55. Furukawa TA, Harai H, Hirai T, et al. Social Support Questionnaire among psychiatric patients with various diagnoses and normal controls. Soc Psychiatry Psychiatr Epidemiol 1999;34(4):216–22.

56. Cohen S, Hoberman HM. Positive events and social supports as buffers of life change stress. J Appl Soc Psychol 1983;13(2):99–125.

57. Cohen S, Mermelstein R, Kamarck T, et al. Measuring the functional components of social support. In: Sarason BR, Sarason IG, editors. Social support: theory, research, and applications. The Hague, The Netherlands: Martinus Nijhoff; 1985. p. 73–94.

58. Boschen KA, Tonack M, Gargaro J. The impact of being a support provider to a person living in the community with a spinal cord injury. Rehabil Psychol 2005;50(4):397–407.

59. Smith TW, Ruiz JM, Uchino BN. Mental activation of supportive ties, hostility, and cardiovascular reactivity to laboratory stress in young men and women. Health Psychol 2004;23(5):476–85.

60. Turner-Cobb JM, Sephton SE, Koopman C, et al. Social support and salivary cortisol in women with metastatic breast cancer. Psychosom Med 2000; 62(3):337–45.

61. Cutrona C, Russell D, Rose J. Social support and adaptation to stress by the elderly. Psychol Aging 1986;1(1):47–54.

62. Weiss RS. Loneliness: the experience of emotional and social isolation. Cambridge (MA): The MIT Press; 1973. p. 236.

63. Blaney NT, Goodkin K, Feaster D, et al. A psychosocial model of distress over time in early HIV-1 infection: the role of life stressors, social support and coping. Psychol Health 1997;12(5):633–53.

64. Elliott TR, Herrick SM, Witty TE, et al. Social support and depression following spinal cord injury. Rehabil Psychol 1992;37(1):37–48.

65. Drageset S, Lindstrom TC. Coping with a possible breast cancer diagnosis: demographic factors and social support. J Adv Nurs 2005;51(3):217–26.

66. Karnell LH, Christensen AJ, Rosenthal EL, et al. Influence of social support on health-related quality of life outcomes in head and neck cancer. Head Neck 2007;29(2):143–6.

67. Canty-Mitchell J, Zimet GD. Psychometric properties of the multidimensional scale of perceived social support in urban adolescents. Am J Community Psychol 2000;28(3):391–400.

68. Clara IP, Cox BJ, Enns MW, et al. Confirmatory factor analysis of the multidimensional scale of perceived social support in clinically distressed and student samples. J Pers Assess 2003;81(3):265–70.

69. Barrera M, Sandler IN, Ramsay TB. Preliminary development of a scale of social support: studies on college students. Am J Community Psychol 1981;9(4):435–47.

70. Lubben JE. Assessing social networks among elderly populations. Fam Community Health 1988; 11(3):42–52.

71. Lubben JE, Gironda MW. Measuring social networks and assessing their benefits. In: Phillipson C, Allan G, Morgan D, editors. Social networks and social exclusion: sociological and policy issues. Hants (UK): Ashgate Publishing Ltd; 2003. p. 20–34.

72. Lubben J, Blozik E, Gillmann G, et al. Performance of an abbreviated version of the Lubben Social Network Scale among three European community-dwelling older adult populations. 2006. Gerontologist 2006;46(4):503–13.

73. Levy-Storms L, Lubben JE. Network composition and health behaviors among older Samoan women. J Aging Health 2006;18(6):814–36.

74. Lehman AF. Instruments for measuring quality of life in mental disorders. I: up to 1996. New York: John Wiley & Sons Ltd; 2006.

75. Katschnig H, Freeman H, Sartorius N. Quality of life in mental disorders. 2nd edition. New York: John Wiley & Sons Ltd; 2006. p. 351.

76. Weissman MM, Bothwell S. Assessment of social adjustment by patient self-report. Arch Gen Psychiatry 1976;33(9):1111–5.

77. Jaycox LH, Marshall GN, Schell T. Use of mental health services by men injured through community violence. Psychiatr Serv 2004;55(4):415–20.

78. Miranda J, Cooper LA. Disparities in care for depression among primary care patients. J Gen Intern Med 2004;19(2):120–6.

79. Dougall AL, Ursano RJ, Posluszny DM, et al. Predictors of posttraumatic stress among victims of motor vehicle accidents. Psychosom Med 2001;63(3):402–11.

80. McNally RJ. Psychological mechanisms in acute response to trauma. Biol Psychiatry 2003;53(9): 779–86.

81. Cohen S, Kamarck T, Mermelstein R. A global measure of perceived stress. J Health Soc Behav 1983;24(4):385–96.

# Collaborative Care Interventions in General Trauma Patients

Megan Petrie, BA, Douglas Zatzick, MD*

**KEYWORDS**

- Collaborative care • PTSD • Trauma center • Alcohol

Every year, approximately 37 million individuals visit American emergency departments because of traumatic injuries.[1] Motor vehicle accidents, violent physical trauma, and other natural or man-made disasters are among the many leading causes of patients visiting acute care medical centers. Of those entering acute care hospital facilities, 2.5 million have sustained injuries severe enough to require inpatient treatment.[1–3]

Physical injury as a result of a traumatic event increases the risk for experiencing psychiatric symptoms, including depression and posttraumatic stress disorder (PTSD), other psychosomatic symptoms, or those without any known medical cause.[4–17] In an analysis of data from the National Study on the Costs and Outcomes of Trauma (NSCOT), the largest study to date assessing functional and work outcomes after an injury, researchers found that 23% of injury survivors were continuing to experience PTSD symptoms a year postinjury.[18] In addition, research indicates that between 20% and 50% of patients with trauma on surgical wards fit the criteria for current or long-term substance abuse.[19,20]

An estimated 10% to 40% of patients presenting to acute medical centers after a physical injury develop symptoms associated with PTSD.[8,11,15,16,21,22] In a 2007 study, Wong and colleagues[23] worked with facial trauma survivors to assess acute care needs and psychiatric symptoms postinjury. Through psychiatric assessments, 34% of study participants showed symptoms of PTSD and 35% expressed symptoms of depression. Similar to other trauma survivors, although these patients expressed interest in treatment for their symptoms, they were unsure where to find treatment, and no patient actually sought out mental health treatment after leaving the acute care facility.

## DELIVERING MENTAL HEALTH CARE AS PART OF TRAUMA CARE SYSTEMS

Survivors of mass trauma, including those injured during the September 11, 2001 terrorist attacks, are at an increased risk for developing psychiatric symptoms after an injury. Guidelines now suggest mental health screenings for patients coming into acute care facilities from a mass trauma or natural disaster.[24] Other identified risk factors for the development of PTSD include prior PTSD trauma with related symptoms, female gender, higher initial heart rate at emergency department arrival, and initial distress after injury.[8,11,17,25–30]

In trauma care systems, patients often receive aftercare that is fragmented between the hospital's follow-up clinics and their primary care providers, with few to no services offered onsite to bridge this gap.[13,31,32] Patients see several providers in a variety of contexts: hospital aftercare, rehabilitation, mental health services, and primary care medicine without a connecting source. Also, many patients leave the emergency department or inpatient ward without an established or referred primary care provider,

Supported by grants K08 MH01610 and R01MH073613 from the National Institute of Mental Health.
Department of Psychiatry and Behavioral Sciences, University of Washington, Seattle, Box 359911, 325 Ninth Avenue, Seattle, WA 98104-2499, USA
* Corresponding author.
*E-mail address:* dzatzick@u.washington.edu

compounding the disconnect between physical and mental health care.[14,33]

The Institute of Medicine (IOM) has developed quality-of-care criteria designed to assist in assessment and intervention of patients with trauma. All patient aftercare should be based on evidence-based practices. In addition to evidence-based practice, health care centers should also ensure that care is equal but client-centered. Patients entering trauma centers come from a heterogeneous population of varying backgrounds, ethnicities, and socioeconomic statuses. The IOM report suggests that patients should receive the same quality of care while still receiving resources that will meet their specific needs. Patients' needs, values, and opinions should be considered when making medical decisions. Patient care should also be continuous, extending to after discharge during follow-up appointments at clinics and rehabilitation centers. The center of care is based on the relationship between the provider(s) and patients. Lastly, the IOM emphasizes the need for collaborative care among health care centers and providers when actively sharing information and plans for aftercare.[34]

However, with current standards of practice at acute care facilities, few patients receive mental health evaluations or treatment even though more than 50% of trauma survivors experience high levels of emotional distress associated with PTSD, depression, and substance use disorders and experience symptoms while on the ward.[15] Patients rarely seek out mental health services on their own after hospital discharge.[35–38] Therefore, although there are many evidence-based interventions available for patients with PTSD symptoms, these are rarely practiced with trauma patients postinjury.

Even with existing trauma interventions in acute care centers, previous studies have experienced difficulty keeping many patients engaged after discharge from the hospital.[39–43] Commonly expressed patient concerns at the time of hospital discharge include physical, financial, and social concerns, and these can interrupt the focus on postinjury psychiatric care.[44] Intervention protocols that assist patients in addressing these concerns seem to allow patients to focus more on any needed psychiatric treatment.[15,44]

## PTSD AND FUNCTIONAL IMPAIRMENT AFTER INJURY

Several studies have shown that PTSD limits independent functioning and quality of life after a physical injury further than physical limitations alone.[16,26,45,46] Zatzick and colleagues recently completed the analysis of the National Study on Costs and Outcomes of Trauma in which the associations between PTSD and functional impairment were examined. Functional outcomes assessed were activities of daily living, health status, and return to major activities, including work. Previously employed patients showing symptoms of either PTSD or depression had a 3-fold increase in odds of not returning to work postinjury. Patients experiencing symptoms of PTSD and depression had 5 to 6 odds increase in not returning to work after their injury when compared with previously employed patients not experiencing any PTSD or depressive symptoms.

Ramchand and colleagues[47] found that physical functioning and PTSD symptoms can have a negative effect on each other in the months after injury. Patients with more severe physical injury expressed greater psychological distress in the months after injury. Likewise, patients with higher levels of PTSD-related symptoms immediately after their injury subsequently experienced more functional impairment.

## DEVELOPING COLLABORATIVE INTERVENTIONS IN GENERAL SURGICAL SETTINGS

As discussed in the introduction, injured patients within acute care facilities are at high risk for developing PTSD and alcohol-use disorders. As is true for many Americans with psychiatric disorders, many patients suffering from PTSD and other psychiatric disorders receive fragmented care postinjury and are not engaged in mental health services at strategic posttrauma points.[48,49]

Previous research has emphasized the important role that collaborative care plays in patients with continuous and comorbid conditions and in integrating patient input on follow-up care and treatment for these conditions.[50,51] Studies have shown efficacy using these collaborative care interventions on patients with depression and anxiety.[50,52–54]

Just as collaborative care interventions have incorporated primary care providers into the provision of mental health services, the introduction of early collaborative care interventions in trauma care systems may serve to integrate acute care providers into posttraumatic mental health care delivery. Using randomized effectiveness designs rooted in the structure, process, and outcome model of intervention delivery, mental health services researchers have demonstrated that combined, collaborative care interventions can improve symptomatic outcomes for patients with depressive and anxiety disorders who are treated in primary care. Collaborative care interventions in primary care settings have sought to find the optimal roles for primary care physicians, nurse practitioners, and mental health specialists in the delivery of care for patients with psychiatric disorders and chronic conditions. Collaborative care interventions hold promise for the delivery of mental health interventions in acute care, because they can incorporate frontline trauma center providers, such as social workers and nurses, into early mental health services delivery and can link trauma center care to outpatient services.

For patients with both mental health concerns and other ongoing medical conditions, the collaborative care model seeks to provide the best care possible from all participating providers, thus incorporating the expertise from these providers in issues relating to their specific field. Providers and the patient should work in conjunction for developing postinjury treatment planning and goals and identifying and providing ideal medical treatment that corresponds with patient needs as well as care for PTSD symptoms, including evidence-based cognitive behavioral therapy treatment and psychopharmacologic methods.

Another key issue in the collaborative care model is the maintenance of the long-term relationship with the patient. This usually falls to the mental health providers who are continuously working with the patients on PTSD symptoms, possible alcohol or substance abuse, and other postinjury life stressors, as well as working with the patient and other providers to maintain continuity of care. The team works with the patient to understand the importance of many postinjury decisions, especially regarding treatment, and to develop the best plan of action.

In their study on patients with facial trauma, Wong and colleagues[23] found numerous patient-perceived obstacles to receiving postinjury mental health treatment, including lack of knowledge concerning where to find services, cost of treatment, and other practical matters, such as lack of transportation. The study results suggest that collaborative care efforts, which are individualized to a patient's specific needs, may assist in overcoming many of these obstacles (including monetary, legal, and other concerns) while also providing the patient with mental health treatment. The collaborative care model not only allows patients to receive mental health treatment but also provides resources that assist in addressing other patient concerns including legal and financial issues.

Many previous studies show that several patients experiencing PTSD symptoms report a decrease in symptoms in the year after their injury.[17,55,56] Therefore, a stepped-care approach that progresses from simpler first-line treatment to more intensive treatments would be most beneficial. The progression to more resource-intensive care could be reserved for patients who initially receive low-level care or no care after injury and do not experience a spontaneous recovery with their symptoms. During the course of the year after their injury, patients would receive an increase in services and intervention based on their specific needs. This would also allow equitable service and care to all patients initially after an injury, despite the lack of mental health resources that many acute care facilities experience.

## PILOTING PATIENT-CENTERED COLLABORATIVE INTERVENTIONS FOR PHYSICALLY INJURED TRAUMA SURVIVORS

Collaborative care interventions for the treatment of the physically injured in general trauma settings seem promising. The rationale and design of an initial pilot study of collaborative patient-centered care was strongly influenced by the results of Gentilello and colleagues'[57] intervention at Harborview. They demonstrated that brief patient-centered counseling provided by a PhD-level clinician in a trauma setting can be useful in helping injured patients explore and reduce their alcohol use after the injury and also reduce the risk of secondary injuries. The initial collaborative care pilot sought to establish the feasibility of having 3 trauma center providers deliver a brief early intervention that aimed to reduce PTSD symptoms.[58] One interventionist was a trauma surgery nurse practitioner with more than a decade of experience as a frontline provider with the trauma surgery service; 2 interventionists were MD consultation liaison psychiatrists. These providers were trained in a case management procedure that aimed to engage injured trauma survivors by providing readily accessible, continuous trauma support in the days and weeks after the injury.

A key component of the trauma support intervention was eliciting, and targeting for improvement, each patient's unique constellation of posttraumatic concerns. Interventionists also received training in brief interventions for PTSD and alcohol use. In accord with a population-based/effectiveness approach, patients were randomly selected from the population of patients admitted to the hospital's Trauma Surgery Service to participate in the study. Only severely brain-injured and non-English-speaking patients were excluded from the investigation. Patients randomly selected for participation in the study had moderate levels of

PTSD symptoms and substance-related comorbidity.

Patients in the intervention group, when compared with controls, manifested significantly decreased PTSD symptom levels at 1 month (P<.05) but not at 4 months after the injury.[58] Examination of the interventionists' logs revealed that patients were engaged in the early intervention and that 75% of patient-interventionist contact occurred between the hospital admission and the 1-month telephone follow-up interview. Interventionists successfully worked with other acute care providers to integrate the early intervention activities with other aspects of acute care treatment delivery (eg, pain control, discharge planning). However, the trauma center–based interventionists frequently encountered difficulty transitioning the care of patients to the community.

## LARGER-SCALE RANDOMIZED EFFECTIVENESS TRIALS OF COLLABORATIVE CARE IN GENERAL MEDICAL SETTINGS

After the first pilot trial, a second, larger stepped collaborative care trial (ie, the Harborview pilot) was implemented.[15] The Harborview pilot study tested an early combined intervention that included continuous master's-level case management during the first 6 months after injury and evidence-based medication and psychotherapy for PTSD delivered by MD/PhD mental health specialists. As with the pilot study, inclusion criteria for the Harborview pilot remained extremely broad. Patients were screened into the study if they exhibited moderate levels of psychological distress in the surgical ward; patients with current substance use issues were also included in the study.

The goal of the 6-month care management intervention was to engage injured trauma survivors in early intervention and to link these patients to appropriate primary care and community services. The care manager began treatment by meeting the injured patient at the bedside and by eliciting, tracking, and targeting for improvement each patient's unique constellation of posttraumatic concerns. The patient and care manager worked to formulate a comprehensive postinjury care plan. To enhance engagement by encouraging spontaneous patient-initiated contact with the intervention team, the care manager's pager was covered by team members 24 h/d, 7 d/wk.

The care manager aimed to ensure that injured patients were linked to appropriate outpatient primary care and community services. The procedures for collaboration with primary care providers were informed by previous trials of consultation psychiatry interventions for depressive and anxiety disorders in primary care. First, the care manager ascertained whether patients had a regular primary care doctor with whom they could follow-up after discharge from the trauma center. During the initial weeks postinjury, the care manager worked to obtain primary care services for any injured patient who did not have a regular provider. When patients had regular providers, these practitioners were contacted by telephone to discuss the postinjury care plan. If necessary, the care manager helped patients schedule primary care visits and provided reminders of scheduled appointments to facilitate attendance at office visits. Patients who expressed interest in linkage to other community services (eg, low-fee legal clinics, pastoral care services) received assistance with these requests as well. In the later months of the care management intervention (eg, months 3–6), primary care providers were again contacted by telephone by intervention team members to summarize postinjury care and ensure adequate care transfer. For patients started on psychotropic medication, primary care providers were also sent a letter notifying them of the current doses and making recommendations for ongoing prescription and side-effect management. Patients with symptomatic recurrences received stepped-up evidence-based care and/or extension of the care manager during the 6- to 12-month postinjury time period.

At 3 months after the injury, the care manager evaluated each intervention patient for PTSD with the Structured Clinical Interview for Diagnostic and Statistical Manual Disorders. Patients diagnosed with PTSD were referred to the team's MD/PhD providers for the initiation of evidence-based medication and psychotherapy treatment. Team members shared information and deliberated with patients concerning the importance of receiving guideline-level treatments for PTSD symptoms. All patients were given their choice regarding treatment options, and patients could receive either medications or cognitive behavioral therapy or both. The investigation's cognitive behavioral therapist delivered an evidence-based protocol that was derived from prior PTSD efficacy studies. The investigation's psychiatrist performed an initial medication evaluation and initiated guideline concordant pharmacologic treatment. For those electing pharmacotherapy, the psychiatrist would stabilize each patient on an initial course of pharmacotherapy. The psychiatrist would then work with each patient's primary care and community mental health providers to ensure that guideline-level treatment was continued beyond the active study intervention phase.

The master's-level care manager had received prior training in the delivery of motivational interviewing interventions. As with the previous motivational interviewing intervention, an initial 30-minute motivational interviewing intervention was delivered in the surgical ward to patients with current or past histories of alcohol abuse/dependence; motivational interviewing booster sessions were delivered on an as-needed basis to patients with ongoing alcohol abuse and/or drinking behaviors that place them at risk for new injury. For receptive patients, the care manager linked patients to community alcohol services (eg, Alcoholics Anonymous).

Review of intervention logs revealed that the care management procedure effectively engaged 90% of intervention patients. Approximately 50% of intervention patients reported no regular source of primary care services at the time of the surgical ward interview; more than 60% of these patients required that their care be coordinated for follow-up with a primary care provider or other community provider. Successful trauma center–primary care provider linkage by the care manager often required multiple attempts during the months postinjury.

The pilot intervention seemed successful. Regression analyses revealed a significant treatment-group-by-time interaction effect for PTSD. The intervention effect coincided with the initiation of evidence-based medication and psychotherapy interventions for PTSD at the 3-month time point. Post hoc analyses revealed that the significant treatment-group-by-time interaction was due to treatment group differences in the adjusted rates of change in PTSD during the 12-months post injury ($P = .02$).[59]

## FUTURE DIRECTIONS

The American College of Surgeons now requires that level I trauma centers must have on-site alcohol screening and brief intervention services as a requisite for trauma center accreditation.[60] This policy mandate is derived from a series of acute care screening and intervention studies documenting improved outcomes for patients receiving clinical interventions targeting postinjury alcohol consumption. In addition, the latest version of the American College of Surgeons publication *Resources for the Optimal Care of the Injured Patient* has recommended PTSD assessments.[60] Thus, future efforts to refine acute trauma care screening and intervention procedures using collaborative care models have the potential to improve the quality of care provided to injured survivors of individual and mass trauma.

## REFERENCES

1. Bonnie RJ, Fulco CE, Liverman CT, editors. Reducing the burden of injury: advancing prevention and treatment. Washington, DC: National Academy Press; 1999.
2. McCaig LF. National hospital ambulatory medical care survey: 1992 emergency department summary, vol. 245. Hyattsville (MD): National Center for Health Statistics; 1994.
3. Rice DR, MacKenzie EJ, Associates. Cost of injury in the United States: a report to congress. San Francisco (CA): Institute for Health and Aging, University of California, and Injury Prevention Center, Johns Hopkins University; 1989.
4. Engel CC, Liu X, McCarthy BD, et al. Relationship of physical symptoms to posttraumatic stress disorder among veterans seeking care for gulf war-related health concerns. Psychosom Med 2000;62:739.
5. Green MM, McFarlane AC, Hunter CE, et al. Undiagnosed post-traumatic stress disorder following motor vehicle accidents. Med J Aust 1993;159:529–36.
6. Helzer JE, Robins LN, McEvoy L. Post-traumatic stress disorder in the general population. Findings of the epidemiological catchment area survey. N Engl J Med 1987;317:1630.
7. Hoge CW, Castro CA, Messer SC, et al. Combat duty in Iraq and Afghanistan, mental health problems, and barriers to care. N Engl J Med 2004;351:13.
8. Holbrook TL, Hoyt DB, Stein MB, et al. Perceived threat to life predicts posttraumatic stress disorder after major trauma: risk factors and functional outcome. J Trauma 2001;51:287.
9. Katon W, Sullivan M, Walker E. Medical symptoms without identified pathology: relationship to psychiatric disorders, childhood and adult trauma, and personality traits. Ann Intern Med 2001;134:917.
10. Koren D, Norman D, Cohen A, et al. Increased PTSD risk with combat-related injury: a matched comparison study of injured and uninjured soldiers experiencing the same combat events. Am J Psychiatry 2005;162:276.
11. Marshall GN, Schell TL. Reappraising the link between peritraumatic dissociation and PTSD symptom severity: evidence from a longitudinal study of community violence survivors. J Abnorm Psychol 2002;111:626.
12. Ursano RJ, Fullerton CS, Epstein RS, et al. Acute and chronic posttraumatic stress disorder in motor vehicle accident victims. Am J Psychiatry 1999;156:589.
13. Zatzick D. Posttraumatic stress, functional impairment, and service utilization after injury: a public health approach. Semin Clin Neuropsychiatry 2003;8:149.

14. Zatzick D, Grossman D, Russo J, et al. Predicting posttraumatic stress symptoms longitudinally in a representative sample of hospitalized injured adolescents. J Am Acad Child Adolesc Psychiatry 2006;45:1188.

15. Zatzick D, Jurkovich G, Russo J, et al. Posttraumatic distress, alcohol disorders, and recurrent trauma across level 1 trauma centers. J Trauma 2004;57:360.

16. Zatzick D, Jurkovich GJ, Gentilello LM, et al. Posttraumatic stress, problem drinking, and functional outcomes after injury. Arch Surg 2002;137:200.

17. Zatzick D, Kang SM, Muller HG, et al. Predicting posttraumatic distress in hospitalized trauma survivors with acute injuries. Am J Psychiatry 2002;159:941.

18. Zatzick D, Wagner A. Evaluating and treating injured trauma survivors in trauma care systems. In: Litz BT, editor. Early intervention for trauma and traumatic loss. New York: The Guileford Press; 2004. p. 263–83.

19. Li G. Epidemiology of substance abuse among trauma patients. Trauma Q 2000;14:353.

20. Soderstrom CA, Smith GS, Dischinger PC, et al. Psychoactive substance use disorders among seriously injured trauma center patients. J Am Med Assoc 1997;277:1769.

21. Ursano RJ, Bell C, Eth S, et al. Practice guideline for the treatment of patients with acute stress disorder and posttraumatic stress disorder. Am J Psychiatry Suppl 2004;161(Suppl 3):11.

22. Zatzick D, Russo J, Roy-Byrne P, et al. The association between posttraumatic stress disorder and functional impairment: does the evidence support early intervention? In National Institute of Mental Health Division of Services and Intervention Research: evidence in mental health services research conference: what types, how much and then what? Washington, DC, April, 2002.

23. Wong E, Marshall G, Shetty V, et al. Survivors of violence-related facial injury: psychiatric needs and barriers to mental health care. Gen Hosp Psychiatry 2007;29:117.

24. National Institute of Mental Health. Mental health consequences of violence and trauma. Washington, DC: National Institute of Mental Health; 2004.

25. Bryant RA, Harvey AG, Guthrie RM, et al. A prospective study of psychophysiological arousal, acute stress disorder, and posttraumatic stress disorder. J Abnorm Psychol 2000;109:341.

26. Michaels AJ, Michaels CE, Moon CH, et al. Posttraumatic stress disorder after injury: impact on general health outcome and early risk assessment. J Trauma 1999;47:460.

27. Michaels AJ, Michaels CE, Zimmerman MA, et al. Posttraumatic stress disorder in injured adults: etiology by path analysis. J Trauma 1999;47:867.

28. O'Donnell ML, Creamer M, Bryant RA, et al. Posttraumatic disorders following injury: an empirical and methodological review. Clin Psychol Rev 2003; 23:587.

29. Winston FK, Kassam-Adams N, Garcia-Espana F, et al. Screening for risk of persistent posttraumatic stress in injured children and their parents. J Am Med Assoc 2003;290:643.

30. Zatzick D, Russo J, Rivara F, et al. The detection and treatment of posttraumatic distress and substance intoxication in the acute care inpatient setting. Gen Hosp Psychiatry 2005;27:57.

31. Horowitz L, Kassam-Adams N, Bergstein J. Mental health aspects of emergency medical services for children: summary of a consensus conference. Acad Emerg Med 2001;8:1187.

32. Sabin JA, Zatzick D, Jurkovich G, et al. Primary care utilization and detection of emotional distress after adolescent traumatic injury: identifying an unmet need. Pediatrics 2006;117:130.

33. Zatzick D, Simon GE, Wagner AW. Developing and implementing randomized effectiveness trials in general medical settings. Clin Psychol Sci Pract 2006;13:53.

34. Committee on Quality of Health Care in America. Crossing the quality chasm: a new health system for the 21st century. Washington, DC: National Academy Press; 2001.

35. Dunn C, Zatzick D, Russo J, et al. Hazardous drinking by trauma patients during the year after injury. J Trauma 2003;54:707.

36. Jaycox LH, Marshall GN, Schell T. Use of mental health services by men injured through community violence. Psychiatr Serv 2004;55:415.

37. McCarthy ML, MacKenzie EJ, Edwin D, et al. Psychological distress associated with severe lower-limb injury. J Bone Joint Surg Am 2003;85:1689.

38. Wong EC, Schell TL, Marshall GN, et al. Mental health service utilization after physical trauma: the importance of physician referral. Med Care 2009; 47:1077–83.

39. Jack K, Glied S. The public costs of mental health response: lessons from the New York City post-9/11 needs assessment. J Urban Health 2002;79:332.

40. Pitman RK, Sanders KM, Zusman RM, et al. Pilot study of secondary prevention of posttraumatic stress disorder with propranolol. Biol Psychiatry 2002;51:189.

41. Roy-Byrne PP, Russo J, Michelson E, et al. Risk factors and outcome in ambulatory assault victims presenting to the acute emergency department setting: implications for secondary prevention studies in PTSD. Depress Anxiety 2004;19:77.

42. Schwarz ED, Kowalski JM. Malignant memories: reluctance to utilize mental health services after a disaster. J Nerv Ment Dis 1992;180:767.

43. Weisaeth L. Acute posttraumatic stress: nonacceptance of early intervention. J Clin Psychiatry 2001; 62:35.

44. Zatzick D, Kang SM, Hinton WL, et al. Posttraumatic concerns: a patient-centered approach to outcome assessment after traumatic physical injury. Med Care 2001;39:327.

45. Greenspan AI, Kellermann AL. Physical and psychological outcomes 8 months after serious gunshot injury. J Trauma 2002;53:707.

46. Holbrook TL, Anderson JP, Sieber WJ, et al. Outcome after major trauma: 12-month and 18-month follow-up results from the trauma recovery project. J Trauma 1999;46:765.

47. Ramchand R, Marshall GN, Schell TL, et al. Posttraumatic distress and physical functioning: a longitudinal study of injured survivors of community violence. J Consult Clin Psychol 2008;76:668.

48. New Freedom Commission on Mental Health. Achieving the promise: transforming mental health care in America. Rockville (MD): DHHS; 2003.

49. Satcher D. Mental health: a report of the Surgeon General. Rockville (MD): US Department of Health and Human Services; 1999.

50. Katon W, Von Korff M, Lin E, et al. Stepped collaborative care for primary care patients with persistent depression: a randomized trial. Arch Gen Psychiatry 1999;56:1109.

51. Von Korff M, Gruman J, Schaefer J, et al. Collaborative management of chronic illness. Ann Intern Med 1997;127:1097.

52. Katon W, Robinson P, Von Korff MV, et al. A mulitfaceted intervention to improve treatment of depression in primary care. Arch Gen Psychiatry 1996;53:924.

53. Roy-Byrne PP, Katon W, Cowley DS, et al. A randomized effectiveness trial of collaborative care for patients with panic disorder in primary care. Arch Gen Psychiatry 2001;58:869.

54. Unutzer J, Katon W, Callahan CM, et al. Collaborative care management of late-life depression in the primary care setting: a randomized controlled trial. J Am Med Assoc 2002;288:2836.

55. Mayou R, Tyndel S, Bryant B. Long-term outcome of motor vehicle accident injury. Psychosom Med 1997;59:578.

56. Rothbaum B, Foa EB. Exposure therapy for PTSD. PTSD Research Quarterly 1999;10:1.

57. Gentilello LM, Rivera FP, Donovan DM, et al. Alcohol interventions in a trauma center as a means of reducing the risk of injury recurrence. Ann Surg 1999;230:473.

58. Zatzick D, Roy-Byrne P, Russo J, et al. Collaborative interventions for physically injured trauma survivors: a pilot randomized effectiveness trial. Gen Hosp Psychiatry 2001;23:114.

59. Zatzick D, Jurkovich G, Rivara F, et al. A national study of posttraumatic stress disorder, depression, and work and functional outcomes after injury hospitalization. Ann Surg 2008;248:429.

60. American College of Surgeons Committee on Trauma. Resources for the optimal care of the injured patient: 2006. Chicago: American College of Surgeons Committee on Trauma; 2006.

# Salivary Biosensors for Screening Trauma-Related Psychopathology

Vivek Shetty, DDS, Dr Med Dent[a],*, Masaki Yamaguchi, PhD[b]

**KEYWORDS**

- Stress response biomarkers • Neuroendocrine response
- Point-of-care testing • Salivary biosensor

As manifest by the preceding articles, facial injuries can exact a sustained psychological toll in vulnerable patients. Most individuals do recover; however, a distinct subset continues to suffer from the psychological stress of the trauma exposure and develop distress and psychiatric illness or exhibit health risk behaviors, such as substance use, that may increase their risk of reinjury. Despite the adverse impact of posttrauma psychopathology on physical recovery, quality of life, and social and vocational functioning, most individuals who develop these mental health problems are not identified or treated early on. A growing body of research indicates that early identification of maladaptive stress reactions provides opportunities for initiating preemptive and targeted mental health interventions. Researchers such as Noy and colleagues[1] have suggested that mental health interventions in the early stages may prevent the crystallization of abnormal stress reactions into entrenched psychiatric sequelae. However, the clinical challenge is one of differentiating between transient distress and precursors of recalcitrant psychiatric sequelae. Existing psychological screening strategies tend to be time- and resource-intensive, and are often not compatible with fast-paced trauma care. Even those clinicians and health care systems interested in providing integrated care to patients with facial injury face decisions on how best to distribute limited resources in an era of growing budgetary constraints. Which patients will need additional psychosocial services, what will be the nature of these services, and when and how will they be provided? Practical and brief screening strategies that facilitate early identification and targeted interventions will go far in directing limited health care resources to those least likely to recover without extensive professional support.

Beyond these logistical and budgetary constraints, the development of collaborative trauma care practices suffer from a lack of training in eliciting information about psychosocial issues or surgeon attitudes about collecting data seemingly unrelated to the restitution of the physical injury.[2] Unlike the swelling, bruising, and radiographic findings that signal a bone fracture, the signs and symptoms of maladaptive stress reactions and ensuing substance use disorders are more subjective and are characterized by a vast range of behaviors. These challenges were evident in the authors' research study,[3] which determined that oral and maxillofacial surgery residents treating facial injury patients did not identify alcohol use in 42% or drug use in more than 65% of individuals with substance use behaviors. Current screening

This work was supported by Grants Nos. 5UO1DA023815 and 5R01DA016850 from the National Institutes of Health/NIDA.

[a] Section of Oral and Maxillofacial Surgery, 23-009 UCLA School of Dentistry, University of California, 10833 Le Conte Avenue, Los Angeles, CA 90095-1668, USA

[b] Department of Welfare Engineering, Faculty of Engineering, Iwate University, 4-3-5 Ueda, Morioka City, 020-8551, Japan

* Corresponding author.

*E-mail address:* vshetty@ucla.edu

Oral Maxillofacial Surg Clin N Am 22 (2010) 269–278

doi:10.1016/j.coms.2010.01.004

practices are unreliable because they rely exclusively on patient self-reports and subjective interviewer assessments of psychopathology. The problem is further compounded by the burdens of interpreting the screening results. Without objective help, clinicians have only their judgment to resolve their clinical impressions, all of which needs to be accomplished in a trauma care setting with other competing agendas and demands. Thus, it is evident that the provision of comprehensive care for patients with orofacial injuries suffers greatly from a lack of objective adjuncts and decision-aid tools to complement the clinical evaluation.

This article addresses meeting the need for practical, standardized, and reliable screening strategies through promising developments in the use of stress response biomarkers and biosensing technology.

## PSYCHOBIOLOGY OF THE TRAUMATIC STRESS RESPONSE

Based on the knowledge that the stimulus of the traumatic stressor precipitates a series of compensatory mechanisms expressed as discernible physiologic changes, increasing attention has focused on identifying and measuring the corresponding biologic indicators.[4] Characterizing the biologic correlates of normal and abnormal psychological responses to the trauma could be very useful in the identification of emerging psychopathology and in directing referrals and treatment. Broadly, the stress response to injury is characterized by a complex and counterbalancing set of hormonal responses in the 2 arms of the neuroendocrine system: the sympathetic nervous system (SNS) and the hypothalamic-pituitary-adrenal (HPA) axis. Immediately after a traumatic stressor, the SNS responds by triggering the adrenal glands to release epinephrine and the sympathetic nerves to squirt out the epinephrine-like chemical norepinephrine all over the body: nerves that wire the heart, salivary glands, gut, and skin. The sympathetic stress response increases the heart rate, blood pressure, and blood glucose levels in muscles and vital organs to help the body adapt to the increased demand. The HPA axis response to the stressor is slower (ie, minutes) and marked by an increase in the release of corticotrophin releasing hormone (CRH) and other neuromodulators from the hypothalamus. CRH stimulates the anterior pituitary gland to release adrenocorticotrophin hormone (ACTH), which in turn stimulates the adrenal glands to release cortisol as well as dehydroepiandosterone (DHEA) and its metabolite (DHEA-S).

Cortisol has an important role in shutting down sympathetic activation and suppressing the HPA axis through a negative feedback mechanism. The antiglucocorticoid properties of DHEA-S are believed to contribute to an upregulation of HPA axis responses as well as mitigate possible deleterious effects of high cortisol levels on the brain.[5] Once the perception of threat recedes, the negative feedback mechanisms help restore hormone levels to baseline. However, if the stressors are extreme or chronic, the homeostatic process may become dysregulated and provoke the altered neuroendocrine patterns associated with various psychopathological conditions.[6] Considerable evidence shows a link between neuroendocrine dysregulation and psychopathology, including mood and anxiety disorders.[7,8]

## SALIVA AS A SOURCE OF STRESS BIOMARKERS

The centrality of hormonal "stress mediators" to normal and maladaptive stress responses renders them an attractive means of connecting the stress experience with the individual's psychobiological response to trauma. However, the intrusiveness and logistical limitations inherent to the pervasive use of blood and urine as sources of peripheral biomarkers have led to the growing interest in the use of saliva as an alternative (see review by Wong[9]). A virtual mirror of the body, saliva can reflect practically the entire spectrum of normal and disease states, including tissue levels of natural substances as well as hormonal and immunologic status.[10] The 3 major salivary glands (parotid, submandibular, and sublingual) and numerous minor glands produce ample amounts (500–1500 mL) of saliva daily.[11] For patients, supplying a saliva sample evokes less anxiety than providing a blood sample, and less embarrassment than producing a urine specimen. For clinicians and laboratory technicians, saliva poses much less risk of exposure to pathogens such as human immunodeficiency virus or hepatitis than blood tests. Unless visibly contaminated with blood, human saliva is not considered a class II biohazard (US Centers for Disease Control), affording researchers and institutions both administrative and safety benefits. Unlike the phlebotomy skills required for blood collection, saliva samples are easily procured. Multiple sampling over the day or over many days can be readily completed in the field or at home, thus increasing the feasibility of doing longitudinal studies.[12] Saliva requires minimal manipulation because it does not clot, and raises fewer ethical concerns than more invasive methods. Furthermore, saliva samples can be obtained without difficulty from children[13] and individuals with physical or mental handicaps.[14] The noninvasive collection of saliva is particularly advantageous when subjects require regular monitoring with repeated sampling. In summary, saliva is an ideal biofluid for biomarker discovery and profiling of mental health disorders and is a promising basis for inexpensive, noninvasive, and easy-to-use diagnostic technology.

## PUTATIVE SALIVARY STRESS BIOMARKERS

The search for salivary indices of the individual stress response has involved various components of the human salivary proteome including cortisol, DHEA-S, testosterone, catecholamines, immunoglobulin A (IgA), and chromogranin-A. Much of the attention of stress researchers has focused on salivary cortisol as an expression of HPA axis activation.[15–17] Assessment of cortisol levels is compounded by a natural diurnal variation: cortisol levels are high in the morning and low at night. Cortisol is thought to enter saliva by passive diffusion and correlates closely with the free physiologically active serum cortisol fraction.[18] Unlike cortisol, conjugated steroid DHEA-S enters saliva via ultrafiltration through the tight junctions between acinar cells and has a serum-saliva correlation of 0.86 (Salimetrics assay). Salivary testosterone levels are significantly correlated ($r = 0.71$) with serum testosterone levels in men, and stressors tend to decrease the testosterone levels.[19] This inverse relationship between stress and testosterone levels was substantiated independently by Opstad[20] and Morgan and colleagues[21] in soldiers participating in military endurance training courses.

Because salivary catecholamines are poorly correlated with plasma concentrations, these catecholamines are not considered as useful indexes of general sympathetic tone.[22] An attractive alternative biomarker of adrenergic stimulation is salivary α-amylase (sAA). Mostly synthesized by the serous acinar cells of the parotid gland, amylase is one of the principal salivary proteins and accounts for 10% to 20% of the total salivary gland-produced protein content. Salivary glands are innervated by both sympathetic and parasympathetic nerves and secrete sAA in response to neurotransmitter stimulation.[23] Several investigators have demonstrated that sAA concentrations are closely associated with plasma catecholamine levels, particularly norepinephrine (NE), and are highly correlated with NE changes in response to stress.[24,25] Numerous studies have shown that sAA levels increase under various physical and psychological stressors.[26–29] Also, sAA levels were found to respond to psychological stress[30–33] or relaxation interventions.[34,35] Salivary chromogranin-A, coreleased with serum catecholamines, has also been investigated as an alternative indicator of the psychosomatic stress response.[36] Yet other researchers have attempted to link salivary IgA (SIgA) levels with the psychological reaction. Tsujita and Morimoto[37] showed that SIgA levels vary temporally with the stress response—high in the acute stress phase and decreased in the presence of chronic stress. Whether these salivary proteins occur as a consequence of the psychological distress or are etiopathological to the stress reactions, it is increasingly evident that they are part of the biologic substrate of psychological disorders. Linking these putative biomarkers to various trauma-related psychopathologies (biomarker qualification) through prospective clinical studies could greatly facilitate integrated care of injured patients.

## "POINT-OF-USE" MEASUREMENT OF SALIVARY STRESS INDICATORS

Salivary biomarkers could play an essential role in trauma care by providing useful information about the patient's psychological condition, supporting treatment decision-making, and helping to understand the mechanisms and evolution of adverse mental health sequelae. The promise of salivary stress biomarkers notwithstanding, their clinical utility has been restricted by the lack of appropriate technology platforms that allow near "real-time" detection and quantification of these biologic response indicators. Integrating early identification, risk stratification, and facilitated referrals of injured patients with maladaptive stress reactions will require that the care providers have timely access to salivary stress biomarker data. Typically, biologic samples collected by patients are processed in centralized laboratories, which results in extended reporting times and is fraught with several potential quality failure points. For example, the total process to deliver a salivary test result involves the multiple steps of sample acquisition, labeling, freezing, transportation, processing in the laboratory (centrifugation of the sample, sorting, aliquoting, loading into analyzer), analysis, and results reporting. The costs associated with expensive analytical equipment and testing supplies, sample acquisition and transport supplies, as well as all the labor costs incurred across the total process can be significant impediments to routine use of salivary biomarkers. Finally, the relative stability of a particular biomarker can dramatically affect the measured levels over the collection-measurement-reporting cycle.

In contrast, the utility of point-of-care (POC) testing of saliva resides in the immediacy of the results reporting. The ability to readily measure salivary stress biomarkers at the site of patient care increases the likelihood that the data will be used by the care provider to inform clinical decision-making and provide appropriate referrals. Moreover, the operating advantages of such POC instrumentation will greatly facilitate future validation studies of putative salivary stress biomarkers. Developments in biosensing technology by the authors' research group now allow the fabrication of versatile biosensing platforms[38] for low-cost, point-of-use devices that can measure and profile putative salivary correlates of the stress response.[39–43] Cheaper, smaller, faster, and smarter POC devices have increased the use of POC approaches by making them cost-effective for many diseases. Embedded system software processes measurable biochemical signals into simple digital feedback displays readily accessible to even nonspecialists.

## SALIVARY BIOSENSORS AS SCREENING TOOLS

In its very essence, a salivary biosensor is a small, self-contained device that uses biologic reactions for detecting and measuring a particular substance (analyte) of interest. The biosensor consists of a biologic recognition element (interacting with the target analyte) in intimate contact with a transducer that translates the biorecognition event into a useful electrical signal. The commonly used transducers include optical, electrochemical, or mass-sensitive elements and generate light, current, or frequency signals, respectively. Depending on the nature of the recognition event, the biosensing platform may be either bioaffinity or biocatalytic. Bioaffinity devices rely on the selective binding of the target analyte to a surface-confined capture element (eg, antibody, oligonucleotide). Biocatalytic devices, in contrast, use an immobilized enzyme for recognizing the target substrate. When exposed to a saliva sample, the interaction of the analyte with the bioreceptor produces a detectable effect that is measured by the transducer and converted into a measurable output such as an electrical signal. The strength of the electrical signal is proportional to the level of the single analyte or group of analytes, and the result is provided on an optical display. **Fig. 1** illustrates the conceptual principle of the biosensing process. Depending on the biomarker of interest, the biosensing platform may use antigen/antibody binding, nucleic acid interactions, or enzymatic interactions to recognize the analyte. The more common forms of transducers tend to use optical detection (luminescence, absorption, surface plasmon resonance, and so forth) or electrochemical detection methods.

**Table 1** and **Fig. 2** summarize the underlying principles of sensor devices used for the detection of salivary biomarkers. The complexities and specificities of the biosensing process increase in the following order: enzymatic methods, antigen-antibody methods, and hybridization methods, while the cost of the tests increases correspondingly. The increasing availability of enzyme-linked immunosorbent assay (ELISA) kits for measuring a range of salivary analytes (eg, Salimetrics LLC, PA, USA) has led to resurgence in the interest in salivary stress biomarkers. Gold colloid-based methods such as localized surface plasmon resonance (LSPR, see **Fig. 2**A) allow for low-cost qualitative tests manifesting the color reactions of ELISA as a visible line on a biochip. Similarly,

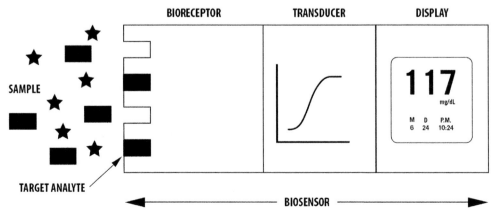

**Fig. 1.** Components of a typical biosensor.

**Table 1**
**Principles of biosensor detection**

| Biologic Recognition Element | Biomarker | Sensor Device |
|---|---|---|
| Enzymatic | Enzyme substrate | Test paper (dry chemistry) |
| | | Enzyme sensor (electrochemical sensor) |
| Immunoassay | Antigen and antibody | ELISA |
| | Hormone | Gold colloid method (LSPR) |
| | Neurotransmitter | Electrophoresis |
| | Enzyme | Immunosensor (electrochemical sensor) |
| | Xenobiotics | SPR |
| Hybridization | mRNA, DNA | DNA chip |

*Abbreviations:* ELISA, enzyme-linked immunosorbent assay; (L)SPR, (localized) surface plasmon resonance.

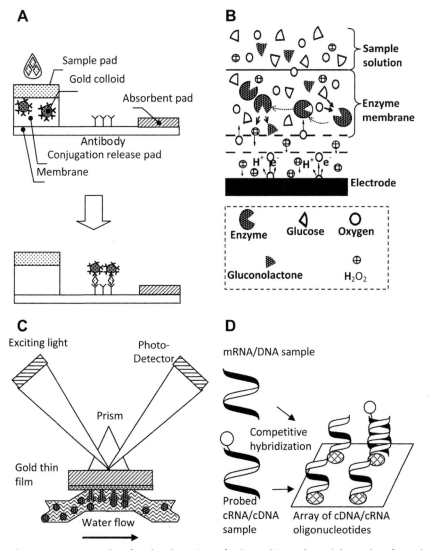

**Fig. 2.** Various biosensing approaches for the detection of salivary biomarkers. (*A*) Local surface plasmon resonance. (*B*) Enzyme sensor. (*C*) Surface plasmon resonance. (*D*) DNA chip.

enzyme sensors (see **Fig. 2**B), immunosensors, and surface plasmon resonance (SPR, see **Fig. 2**C) display the color reactions of the ELISA process by way of electrochemical or optical phenomena, and thus allow measurements that are both highly sensitive and continuous. The DNA chip (DNA microarray) is a relatively new tool used to identify mutations in genes. The DNA chip, which consists of a small glass plate encased in plastic, is manufactured in a manner similar to a computer microchip (see **Fig. 2**D). The surface of each chip can contain thousands of short, synthetic, single-stranded DNA sequences. When the chip is exposed to a biofluid, competitive hybridization occurs between the immobilized synthetic cDNA/cRNA strands and mRNA/DNA in the sample. Radioactive or fluorescence tagging makes automatic detection possible. Because chip technology is still relatively new, it is presently only used as a research tool.

To realize the diagnostic promise of salivary biomarkers for identifying patients at risk for psychopathology after traumatic exposure, the authors have been developing hand-held, POC biosensors that can be used in various acute care settings. The design challenge was to develop a low-cost biosensor whose operation is simple and robust enough to deliver laboratory accuracy and reliability in locations far less well controlled than the laboratory. Because the early adrenergic response has been implicated in the development of traumatic psychopathology, the authors have focused initially on the measurement of sAA that reflects SNS activity. Their biosensor system design uses an inexpensive ($\approx$ \$1), disposable plastic saliva collection strip, and a hand-held reader (**Fig. 3**).

Briefly, the saliva collector at the tip of the test strip is placed under the tongue, allowed to saturate with saliva ($\approx$ 10 seconds), and inserted into the reader. This act activates the reader and initiates a transfer of the collected saliva onto the biosensing platform where the transferred sAA metabolizes a chromogenic substrate to yield a colored product. The embedded microprocessor (MPU) notes the activation of the reader as the initiation of the reaction time (t = 0 s). At t = 10 seconds, an alarm indicates the end of saliva transfer and the collector/strip is removed from the reader. At t = 20 seconds, the reflectance of the product of the enzyme reaction is measured photometrically and the sAA levels reported on the display along with a date and time stamp. Normalizing equations for temperature ($R^2 = 0.99$) and pH ($R^2 = 0.96$) inputted into the biosensors' MPU minimize the impact of variations in ambient temperature and salivary pH. An embedded miniature thermosensor measures the ambient temperature at the time of saliva collection, and the temperature adjustment equation within the biosensor MPU transforms the measured values into sAA activity at 37°C. The single-use plastic strip, similar to the paper strips for glucose monitoring of diabetics, is based on dry reagents and allows considerable simplification of the analytical system and freedom from complex maintenance, calibration, and quality control procedures.

## PERFORMANCE CHARACTERISTICS OF SALIVARY BIOSENSOR PROTOTYPE

A fundamental quality of any salivary biosensor is its ability to provide reliable analytical results in various field conditions. Thus, verification of the performance characteristics (analytical validation) of a biosensor should include assessment of its accuracy (ie, how closely the biosensor readings compare with a gold standard method) and precision (ie, how reproducible the biosensor measurements are). The authors verified the accuracy of the sAA biosensor prototype by establishing the correspondence between the portable sAA biosensor and the "gold standard"—a conventional, laboratory-based Olympus 400AU clinical chemistry analyzer. Briefly, 20 normal, healthy subjects provided saliva samples by passive drool. The sAA levels in the individual samples were determined using 5 biosensor prototypes and compared with the results of the Olympus analyzer. **Fig. 4** summarizes the consistent readings provided by the individual biosensors and the strong positive correlations ($r = 0.989$) between the sAA biosensor readings and the Olympus analyzer. Fitting a linear regression model predicting biosensor readings from the "gold standard" produced a slope

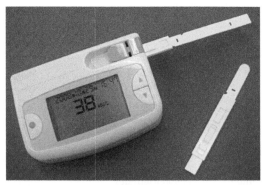

**Fig. 3.** Saliva collection strip and prototype biosensor for point-of-use measurement of salivary alpha-amylase (sAA).

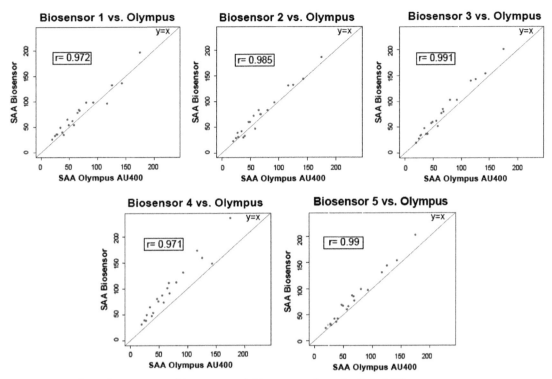

**Fig. 4.** Concordance between sAA biosensors and Olympus analyzer (units in kU/l).

estimate = 1.09 and an $R^2$ = 0.98 (**Fig. 5**). An intraclass correlation coefficient of 0.97 indicated that less than 3% of any measurement variability could be attributable to biosensor. Simply stated, if several the sAA biosensors were deployed in field studies, the measurement variability across the biosensors (ie, the noise) would be minimal when compared with the natural variability in sAA levels in the study population.

Reproducibility of sAA biosensor measurements was evaluated by repeating the analysis of 5 saliva samples after 6 weeks (**Fig. 6**). There was no apparent "drift" in the data as the measurements across the testing points did not appear to differ in their bias, mean, or variation. Thus, based on these biosensor validation studies, it appears the sAA biosensor prototypes are reliable and possess the precision, accuracy, and reproducibility required for routine POC use in trauma settings.

## CLINICAL IMPLICATIONS

The psychological burden of traumatic injury in general, and orofacial injury in particular, provides a compelling rationale for an integrated care approach that addresses all aspects of the recovery process. The use of putative biologic correlates to rapidly identify and differentiate between normal and pathogenic psychological processes has the potential to fundamentally change the way care is delivered to trauma patients. Such an approach would be more reliable, practical, and informative about the pathogenesis and trajectory of maladaptive stress reactions than the existing subjective way of assessing psychopathologic parameters. Surgeons, alerted to evolving morbidity through POC testing of salivary stress biomarkers, would be positioned to make timely treatment decisions and referrals for targeted interventions. A biomarker-based

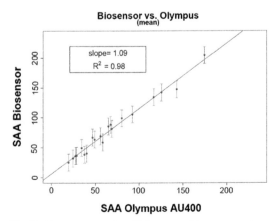

**Fig. 5.** Linear regression fit to mean biosensor values (units in kU/l).

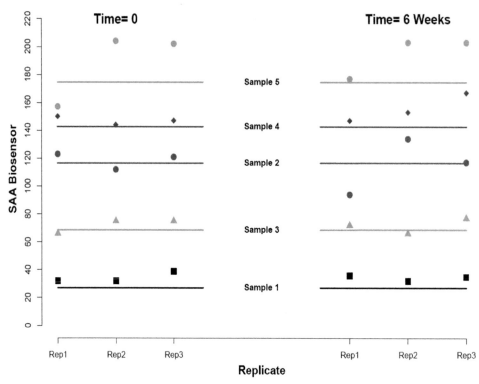

**Fig. 6.** Reproducibility of sAA biosensor verified by repeat measurements of 5 saliva samples. Negligible variation from the "true value" (*horizontal lines* representing the Olympus AU400 readings) indicate minimal measurement drift (units in kU/l).

strategy would also be very useful for tracking disease progression and monitoring response to any treatment. The clinical utility of stress biosensors is predicated on the notion that select salivary biomarkers can serve as indicators of normal or pathogenic processes. An improved awareness of the psychological impact of facial injury could drive the discovery and validation of additional biomarkers for screening psychiatric disorders. Research studies correlating the dynamic alterations of the salivary proteome with the psychological changes related to mental health sequelae will support integrative models for understanding risk and resilience to traumatic psychopathology. The search for peripheral markers of stress to complement clinical evaluation is not unlike biomarker discovery in other specialties such as cardiac transplantation, where overexpression of myocardial proteins such as troponin is used to predict the onset of rejection several weeks prior to conventional histologic diagnosis. Quantitative measurements that provide information about biologic processes will greatly improve the nosology of posttraumatic stress disorders, and help advance the screening, diagnosis,

treatment, and prevention of mental health consequences of violence and trauma.

## FUTURE PERSPECTIVES

The application of a salivary stress biomarker strategy to trauma care hinges on the development of devices and technologies that allow systematic measurement and reporting of target biomarkers. The rapidly evolving disciplines of proteomics, bioengineering, analytical chemistry, and computational biology are producing various new tools and biosensing platforms that are well equipped to monitor the presence or absence of an increasing array of biomarkers. Indeed, some have already been deployed into devices that are already used in clinical settings for the diagnosis or prognosis of certain diseases.[44] The authors' preliminary biosensor development suggests that the measurement and interpretation of salivary proteome levels by hand-held biosensors is a practical, reproducible, less invasive, inexpensive, and point-of-use alternative to the invasive and labor-intensive blood or urine profiling approaches currently used by traumatic stress researchers.

One of the most rapidly advancing of these fronts is the area of multianalyte biosensing, which acknowledges the substantial heterogeneity among psychiatric sequelae and the corresponding inadequacy of a "single biomarker" approach for measuring and tracking severe stress reactions. Future developments in biosensing technologies that allow systematic interrogation of differentially expressed salivary proteins will permit assessment of each psychopathogical response by cross-referencing it to at least 3 neurohormonal markers linked to mental health risk and resilience.[45] The authors anticipate that prospective clinical studies will lead to the development of libraries of executable algorithms and treatment decision trees. Once inputted into the biosensor microprocessor, these algorithms could analyze patterns in salivary stress biomarkers to generate simple feedback displays readily accessible to even nonspecialist personnel. Such "smart systems" will bridge the gaps created by the relative lack of mental health specialists in trauma care settings because the processed output will not require specialized training or knowledge to interpret or implement. Enabled by this technology, surgeons and other health care providers will be able to conduct timely restorative interventions or refer "at-risk" individuals for specialized mental health care to protect against untoward psychiatric reactions. The maturation of the salivary biosensors into commercial devices will happen as the functionality, performance, and production costs improve. In the long term, the authors expect that continuing advances and a growing convergence of proteomic and genomic profiling, biosensing technology, and bioinformatics will create a paradigm shift in the understanding, diagnosis, and management of traumatic stress and psychopathology.

## REFERENCES

1. Noy S, Levy R, Solomon Z. Mental health care in the Lebanon War, 1982. Isr J Med Sci 1984;20:360–3.
2. Chandra A, Marshall GN, Shetty V, et al. Barriers to seeking mental health care after treatment for orofacial injury at a large, urban medical center: concordance of patient and provider perspectives. J Trauma 2008;65(1):196–202.
3. Murphy DA, Shetty V, Resell J, et al. Substance use in vulnerable patients with orofacial injury: prevalence, correlates, and unmet service needs. J Trauma 2009;66(2):477–84.
4. Delahanty DL, Nugent NR. Predicting PTSD prospectively based on prior trauma history and immediate biological responses. Ann N Y Acad Sci 2006;1071:27–40.
5. Rasmusson AM, Vythilingam M, Morgan CA. The neuroendocrinology of posttraumatic stress disorder: new directions. CNS Spectr 2003;8: 651–7.
6. McEwen BS. Allostasis and allostatic load: implications for neuropsychopharmacology. Neuropsychopharmacology 2000;22:108–24.
7. Stratakis CA, Chrousos GP. Neuroendocrinology and pathophysiology of the stress system. Ann N Y Acad Sci 1995;771:1–18.
8. Ehring T, Ehlers A, Cleare AJ, et al. Do acute psychological and psychobiological responses to trauma predict subsequent symptom severities of PTSD and depression? Psychiatry Res 2008; 161(1):67–75.
9. Wong DT. Salivary diagnostics. J Calif Dent Assoc 2006;34(4):283–5.
10. Mandel ID. Salivary diagnosis: more than a lick and a promise. J Am Dent Assoc 1993;124:85–7.
11. Navazesh M, ADA Council on Scientific Affairs and Division of Science. How can oral health care providers determine if patients have dry mouth? J Am Dent Assoc 2003;134:613–20.
12. Holm-Hansen C, Tong G, Davis C, et al. Comparison of oral fluid collectors for use in a rapid point-of-care diagnostic device. Clin Diagn Lab Immunol 2004;11: 909–12.
13. Shimada M, Takahashi K, Ohkawa T, et al. Determination of salivary cortisol by ELISA and its application to the assessment of the circadian rhythm in children. Horm Res 1995;44:213–7.
14. Samuels SC, Furlan PM, Boyce A, et al. Salivary cortisol and daily events in nursing home residents. Am J Geriatr Psychiatry 1997;5:172–6.
15. Yehuda R. Neuroendocrine aspects of PTSD. Handb Exp Pharmacol 2005;169:371–403.
16. Yehuda R. Advances in understanding neuroendocrine alterations in PTSD and their therapeutic implications [review]. Ann N Y Acad Sci 2006; 1071:137–66.
17. Breslau N. Neurobiological research on sleep and stress hormones in epidemiological samples. Ann N Y Acad Sci 2006;1071:221–30.
18. Kirschbaum C, Hellhammer DH. Salivary cortisol in psychoneuroendocrine research: recent developments and applications. Psychoneuroendocrinology 1994;19:313–33.
19. Elman I, Breier A. Effects of acute metabolic stress on plasma progesterone and testosterone in male subjects: relationship to pituitary-adrenocortical axis activation. Life Sci 1997;61:1705–12.
20. Opstad PK. Androgenic hormones during prolonged physical stress, sleep and energy deficiency. J Clin Endocrinol Metab 1992;74:1176–83.
21. Morgan CA 3rd, Wang S, Mason J, et al. Hormone profiles in humans experiencing military survival training. Biol Psychiatry 2000;47(10):891–901.

22. Chiappin S, Antonelli G, Gatti R, et al. Saliva specimen: a new laboratory tool for diagnostic and basic investigation. Clin Chim Acta 2007;383:30–40.
23. Garrett JR. Effects of autonomic nerve stimulations on salivary parenchyma and protein secretion. Front Oral Biol. In: Garrett JR, Ekstrfm J, Anderson LC, editors. Neural mechanisms of salivary gland secretion. Basel (Switzerland): S. Karger AG; 1999. p. 59–79.
24. Kyriacou K, Garrett JR, Gjorstrup P. Structural and functional studies of the effects of sympathetic nerve stimulation on rabbit submandibular salivary glands. Arch Oral Biol 1998;33(4):271–80.
25. Rohleder N, Nater UM, Wolf JM, et al. Psychosocial stress-induced activation of salivary alpha-amylase: an indicator of sympathetic activity? Ann N Y Acad Sci 2004;1032:258–63.
26. Gilman S, Thornton R, Miller D, et al. Effects of exercise stress on parotid gland secretion. Horm Metab Res 1979;11(7):454.
27. Nater UM, Rohleder N, Gaab J, et al. Human salivary alpha-amylase reactivity in a psychosocial stress paradigm. Int J Psychophysiol 2005;55(3):333–42.
28. Nater UM, La Marca R, Florin L, et al. Stress-induced changes in human salivary alpha-amylase activity—associations with adrenergic activity. Psychoneuroendocrinology 2006;31(1):49–58.
29. Nater UM, Gaab J, Rief W, et al. Recent trends in behavioral medicine. Curr Opin Psychiatry 2006;19(2):180–3.
30. Bosch JA, Brand HS, Ligtenberg TJ, et al. Psychological stress as a determinant of protein levels and salivary-induced aggregation of Streptococcus gordonii in human whole saliva. Psychosom Med 1996;58:374–82.
31. Bosch JA, Brand HS, Ligtenberg AJ, et al. The response of salivary protein levels and S-IgA to an academic examination are associated with daily stress. J Psychophysiol 1998;12:384–91.
32. Bosch JA, De Geus EJ, Veerman EC, et al. Innate secretory immunity in response to laboratory stressors that evoke distinct patterns of cardiac autonomic activity. Psychosom Med 2003;65:245–58.
33. Skosnik PD, Chatterton RT, Swisher T, et al. Modulation of attentional inhibition by norepinephrine and cortisol after psychological stress. Int J Psychophysiol 2000;36:59–68.
34. Morse DR, Schacterle GR, Esposito JV, et al. Stress, relaxation and saliva: a follow-up study involving clinical endodontic patients. J Human Stress 1981;7:19–26.
35. Morse DR, Schacterle GR, Zaydenberg M, et al. Salivary volume and amylase activity: I. Relaxation versus relaxed chewing. J Am Soc Psychosom Dent Med 1983;30:85–96.
36. Nakane H. Salivary chromogranin A as an index of psychosomatic stress response. Biomed Res 1998;18:401–6.
37. Tsujita S, Morimoto K. Secretory IgA in saliva can be a useful stress marker. Environ Health Prev Med 1999;4(1):1–8.
38. Yamaguchi M, Kanemaru M, Kanemori T, et al. Flow-injection-type biosensor system for salivary amylase activity. Biosens Bioelectron 2003;18(5–6):835–40.
39. Yamaguchi M, Kanemori T, Kanemaru M, et al. Performance evaluation of salivary amylase activity monitor. Biosens Bioelectron 2004;20(3):491–7.
40. Yamaguchi M, Takeda K, Onishi M, et al. Non-verbal communication method based on a biochemical marker for people with severe motor and intellectual disabilities. J Int Med Res 2006;34(1):30–41.
41. Yamaguchi M, Deguchi M, Wakasugi J, et al. Hand-held monitor of sympathetic nervous system using salivary amylase activity and its validation by driver fatigue assessment. Biosens Bioelectron 2006;21(7):1007–14.
42. Yamaguchi M, Sakakima J. Evaluation of driver stress in a motor-vehicle driving simulator using a biochemical marker. J Int Med Res 2007;35(1):91–100.
43. Takai N, Yamaguchi M, Aragaki T, et al. Gender-specific differences in salivary biomarker responses to acute psychological stress. Ann N Y Acad Sci 2007;1098:510–5.
44. Song S, Xu H, Fan C. Potential diagnostic applications of biosensors: current and future directions [review]. Int J Nanomedicine 2006;1(4):433–40.
45. Charney DS. Psychobiological mechanisms of resilience and vulnerability: implications for successful adaptation to extreme stress [review]. Am J Psychiatry 2004;161(2):195–216.

# Index

*Note:* Page numbers of article titles are in **boldface** type.

## A

Abuse, intimate partner violence, orofacial injuries as markers for, **239–246**
  substance, facial injuries and, **231–238**
Adolescents, substance abuse and facial injury among, 232
Aftercare, psychosocial, after facial injuries, barriers to, **247–250**
    concordance of perspectives on, 249–250
    patient perspectives on, 247–248
    provider perspectives on, 248–249

## B

Barriers, to collaborative care of patients with orofacial injuries, **247–250**
    concordance of provider and patient perspectives, 249–250
    patient perspectives, 247–248
    provider perspectives, 248–249
Biomarkers, salivary biosensors for screening trauma-related psychopathology, **269–278**
    "point of use" measurement of salivary stress indicators, 271–272
    as screening tools, 272–273
    clinical implications, 275–276
    performance characteristics of prototype, 274–275
    psychobiology of traumatic stress response, 270
    putative markers, 271
    saliva as source of stress biomarkers, 270–271

## C

Collaborative care, of patients with facial injuries, 209–278
    as markers for intimate partner violence, **239–246**
    barriers to, **247–250**
      concordance of provider and patient perspectives, 249–250
      patient perspectives, 247–248
      provider perspectives, 248–249
    interventions in general trauma patients, **261–267**
      delivering mental health care as part of trauma care systems, 261–262
      developing interventions in general surgical settings, 262–263

larger scale randomized effectiveness trials in general medical settings, 264–265
      piloting patient-centered collaborative interventions for physically injured trauma survivors, 263–264
      post-traumatic stress disorder and functional impairment after injury, 262
    long-term psychological sequelae of, **217–224**
    psychosocial characteristics and needs of, **209–215**
    salivary biosensors for screening psychopathology related to, **269–278**
    screening for psychiatric problems, **225–229**
    social support and resource needs as mediators of recovery, **251–259**
    substance use and, **231–238**
Complications, of facial injuries related to substance abuse, 233

## D

Demographics, sociodemographic profiles of patients with orofacial injury, 210
Dental schools, curricula to identify risk predictors for injuries related to intimate partner violence, 243–244
Depression, major, screening for, in orofacial trauma setting, 226–228
Domestic violence, orofacial injuries as markers for, **239–246**

## E

Education, dental and medical, curricula to identify risk predictors for injuries related to intimate partner violence, 243–244

## F

Facial injuries, collaborative care of patients with, 209–278
    as markers for intimate partner violence, **239–246**
    barriers to, **247–250**
    interventions in general trauma patients, **261–267**
    long-term psychological sequelae of, **217–224**
    psychosocial characteristics and needs of, **209–215**

Oral Maxillofacial Surg Clin N Am 22 (2010) 279–281
doi:10.1016/S1042-3699(10)00046-4

oralmaxsurgery.theclinics.com

# Moving?

## Make sure your subscription moves with you!

To notify us of your new address, find your **Clinics Account Number** (located on your mailing label above your name), and contact customer service at:

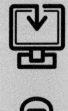

**Email: journalscustomerservice-usa@elsevier.com**

**800-654-2452** (subscribers in the U.S. & Canada)
**314-447-8871** (subscribers outside of the U.S. & Canada)

**Fax number: 314-447-8029**

**Elsevier Health Sciences Division**
**Subscription Customer Service**
**3251 Riverport Lane**
**Maryland Heights, MO 63043**

*To ensure uninterrupted delivery of your subscription, please notify us at least 4 weeks in advance of move.

Printed and bound by CPI Group (UK) Ltd, Croydon, CR0 4YY

03/10/2024

01040344-0016